I0134828

The Yoga Of

Remembrance

By Shivani Howe.

Published by The Living Yoga Society 2018

Copyright © 2018 by Shivani Howe

All rights reserved. This book or any portion thereof may not be reproduced or used in any manner whatsoever without the express written permission of the publisher except for the use of brief quotations in a book review.

Printed in Canada

First Printing, June 2018

Living Yoga Society
Po Box 72
Ta Ta Creek, BC
Canada
V0B2H0

www.livingyogasociety.org

Cover Illustration: Ahimsamurti
Biography Photos: Nicole Leclair
Cover Design: Jason Toner, Big Magic Design

This is the story of how we begin to
Remember,
This is the powerful pulsing of love in the vein,
After the dream of falling and calling your name out,
These are the roots of rhythm,
And the roots of rhythm remain...

Paul Simon - Under African Skies

Dedication:

In humility I offer this book to the lotus feet of Swami Satyananda, Swami Satyasangananda and Swami Niranjanananda of the Saraswati Lineage. There are no words that can properly express my gratitude for the inspiration, support and blessings you have bestowed upon my life. My deepest Pranams. Namo Narayana.

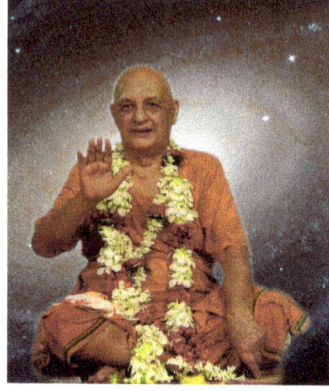

Sri Sw Satyananda
Saraswati (Sri Swamiji)

I offer you a three eyed coconut,
My ego on a platter,
Then I step back with eyes,
Humbly cast,
I beg of you to split it open,
Free me from mayas bind,
Offering my flesh to the hungry,
And my milk to nourish the babes of tomorrow.

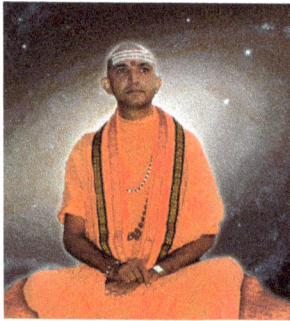

Sw Niranjanananda
Saraswati (Sw Niranjan)

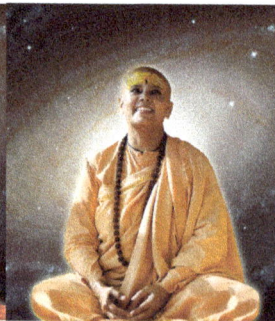

Sw Satyasangananda
Saraswati (Sw Satsangi)

For Narayana Madhu,

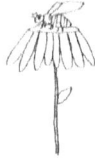

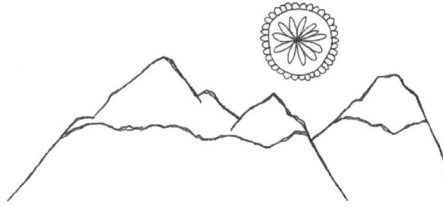

CONTENTS:

Foreword: By Salvatore Zambito   … … … … … … … … … … 2
    Preface: 4
    Acknowledgements: 7

Introduction: 8
Chapter One: Ma Durga Jai Ho   19
Chapter Two: Tabula Rasa   28
Chapter Three: Walking the Walk   34
Chapter Four: Meeting a Master   39
Chapter Five: A Prayer and a Promise - part one   46
Chapter Six: The Bird and the Bees   61
Chapter Seven: Maha Samadhi and the Dream   73
Chapter Eight: This Is How God Speaks   79
Chapter Nine: Wake Up, Surrender, Receive   85
Chapter Ten: The Boon of Vak   88
Chapter Eleven: Foundational Moments   97
Chapter Twelve: The Onion of Indignation   101
Chapter Thirteen: The Illusion of Separateness   108
Chapter Fourteen: A Prayer and a Promise - part two   120

Epilogue: 127
Biography: 128

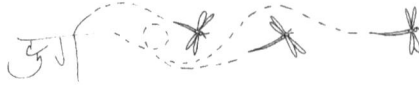

FOREWORD

offered by ∼ Salvatore Zambito

We are told that in the last moments of the Buddha's physical life, he raised himself from his sickbed and looked over his assembled disciples. Lifting his right hand in benediction, he said, "Sammasati," and left the physical world.

"Sammasati," Pali for remember or remembrance.

Gautama, the Buddha, was an expert at spinning riddles to confound the mind. With "Sammasati," he concluded his teaching on this note. "What does he mean, *remembrance?*" his disciples started inquiring immediately.

"He meant to always live in our hearts with the ineffable beauty of moments spent sitting with a Buddha," many confidently asserted.

"He meant for us to always reflect on his teachings and be diligent in the practices he conveyed," others claimed with equal confidence.

"Remembrance itself is a practice," said still others.

The debates ranged to still other opinions.

Finally, someone asked Gautama's senior disciple what his experience of "Sammasati" was. Looking every bit as serene as the Buddha himself, he replied, "Always remember, you are a Buddha."

Our sister Shivani has produced a *Remembrance.*

As a brief autobiographical sketch of her spiritual life to this point in her physical incarnation she covers all the points considered by the disciples of the Buddha after his departure.

Shivani tells of the joy of sitting with her Sat Guru, Sw Satyananda Saraswati. She chronicles her intimate and uncanny communications with Satyananada's senior disciple, Sw Satsangi.

She relates the challenges posed by assigned practices. Satyananda suggests that we break through to deeper states when we are "a little tired". Ha! The general population seems to have the mistaken belief that deep inner peace is an immediate outcome of the first step on the Path. Again, "Ha!". We must resolve every inner conflict before we gain inner peace. Most of all, Shivani shares the deep internal confrontations that are the essence of the genuine spiritual path. Few have the courage and resolution to undertake this relentless self-assessment and often-uncomfortable transmutation. Shivani does.

Taken together, you are holding a story that will take you far from ungrounded spiritual abstractions into the realm usually reserved for action novels and thrillers – except that these adventures are the real thing. With a little luck, Shivani will challenge and inspire you to follow the Path of the Heart and find your own adventures in dimensions and domains not charted in conventional Western society.

Salvatore Zambito
May 29, 2018
Olympic Peninsula,
Washington State; USA

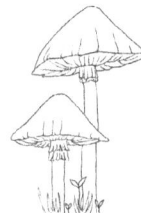

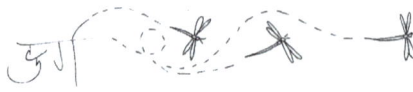

PREFACE

We are a species clouded with amnesia. Spinning in a whirlwind of doing, not realizing that we are here to shed our skin of ignorance, like the snake peels its old casing; not in disgust, but for the Soul purpose of making more room to fill our world with innate and timeless beauty.

This magical life, which is but a spark in Time, launches itself off hindsight, through the eye of now, towards the moving target of hope. It can sometimes feel like you are permanently on spin cycle with soap in your eyes, but as the Ancestors, those who have come before us in this lifetime and the last, have taught us: it is in Remembrance, the reconnecting of our threads, not to the human carcass, but to our Soul nature that is why we have taken our two legged form.

As I look at the tremendous changes my life has gone through in the last 30 something years, I have come to realize that many times during this life, I have been nudged, guided and inspired by forces seen and unseen in ways that swell forth gratitude from the depths of my being. Although I was born and raised in New Zealand, again and again the culture of Mother India, and the wisdom, lineages and traditions She holds for all, have kept showing up in my life. From the first time I donned sari at age 9, to the 12 trips in as many

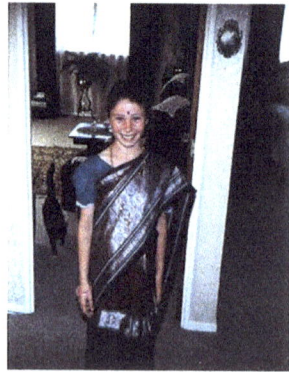

The first time I ever wore a Sari.and the first time Mother India touched my Soul in this lifetime. Navaratri Celebrations aprox 9 years old.

years, I have journeyed to learn at the foot of incredible souls who have climbed the mountain of human potential and are now setting the example for others of how to explore this life from the inside out and to fully embody our potential as Souls having a human experience.

This book is an offering, a declaration, acknowledging the times my personal reality has been touched by direct experiences of the Light and of Grace. How they have impacted my life and how I now call upon them as tools to Remembrance.

I use the word reality, for these stories are my perspective on times and experiences that are incredibly subjective. I do not proclaim my experience of the Soul's mentioned in this book to be anything more than an expression of my own perspective of our interactions. Yet, I share them here, for it is these moments in time that I perceive to be some of the true treasures of my life thus far and it is what it is in these pages that have given me the most solace, faith, and courage to keep stepping forward on this path to living my fullest potential. As Divinity, expressing itself through a spark of the perspective within an individual Soul having a human experience on Earth.

There is a teaching, one that seems to have a somewhat fluid line, of not sharing spiritual experiences or interactions with others as it is sometimes said to disempower the event or cheapen the moment. I understand and respect this perspective from the point that if a story or event of the Divine is used to create separation, conjure the illusion of the person being "special" or "more than another" it can turn the event into an egoic weapon to boost ones own perceived individual importance. However, in my years of reading stories about many different Spiritual Masters and moments of Divine interaction, it is the writers' candid honesty of the moments of unexplainable magic, to the rational mind, that has been a most powerful catalyst in my own heart's opening. These stories were used not to create separation, but inspiration. Comfort that it is not someone who is special that experiences these glimpses, but one who genuinely seeks to know thySelf through the interconnectivity of all being ONE. It was for this reason, when I felt I could no longer put the idea of writing this book to the side, I sought blessings to put these stories to paper.

It is in this vein that I offer this book. A sharing of these kernels of my heart, of my experience of life's magic and Divine wonder in a hope that it will inspire others to prioritize and create their own personal relationship with the Divine and with the Light Bearers, the Gurus that walk the Earth.

Om and Prem

Shivani

18th April 2018
Akshaya Tritiya

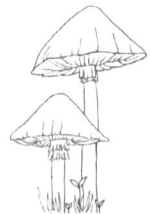

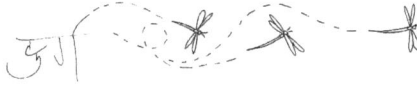

ACKNOWLEDGEMENTS

They say it takes a village to raise a child, and this book, having felt like another child, is no different.

Id like to take this time to offer my heartfelt gratitude to my beloved husband Paramjyoti, and our beautiful son Narayana, for always supporting my crazy artistic endeavours and giving me the encouragement and space to see them through. You are my prayer answered.

To Aradhana, my Editor and partner on this project who's dedication, kindness, and many many selfless hours has kept the momentum going all the way through to this finished offering.

To my Mother for always supporting my artistic side and giving me the encouragement to believe I could do whatever I put my full heart and Soul into.

Anandashakti. my first Yoga teacher, who prepared me to meet my Gurus, and showed me that there was another way to move through this world.

Salvatore and Rebecca Zambito, you are an inspiration and I thank you for all your encouragement and kindness.

To Omshanti and Chaitanya for the endless hours of seva you have offered and continue to offer in the building of 'Niwas and all the support you give in helping us fulfill the vision of having a place for people to come and experience the light of our beloved Sri Swamiji.

To Atmanidhi for your beautiful doodles, and Jess Sculist for your keen eye and kindness.

And to those before me who have had the courage to express the kernels of their hearts in literary form no matter how it "out there" may have seemed to those around them, Martin Pretchel, Dr. Clarissa Pinkola Estés, Stephen Buhner, Rilke, Krishna Das, Ram Das, Khalil Gibran to name but a few.
To all, my heart felt Gratitude.

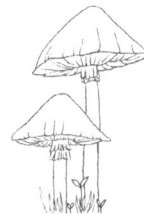

7

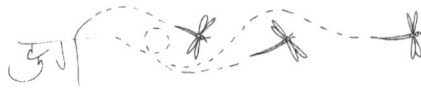

INTRODUCTION

The concepts and teachings in this book are not complex and yet when we use our over functioning, rationalizing and logistical brains to understand them, the deeper meanings and opportunities can too easily get lost. The stories shared here are prefaced by yogic themes and teachings that, I hope, will help bring context from a yogic perspective as to how these moments have shaped my reality. This aspect of the book is food for your mind. The stories are for your heart. They require you to soften your skin and read with your heart, rather than mind, from a soft and expanded perception allowing the words and themes to vibrate within your very core and perhaps touch a part of you that has been dormant. It is my hope that if you are able to receive and digest the stories from that place of dilation that the deepest part of you will attune to a frequency of Remembrance of the essence of your own being.

For this life is magical. Life, is constantly trying to catch our attention to show us a reality we didn't believe could exist just one moment before. Constantly trying to get us to recognize the beauty in the illusion we call reality, so that we may finally recognize, Re-member, the truth of what lies just beyond what we immediately see and feel. That the process of the immediate experience, balanced with seeking to understand "how it was done", leads to an expanded awareness of the event, the cause, the effect and the experience that the whole process has invoked.

The Yoga of Re-membrance is a practice within the heart centered or devotionally orientated path of Bhakti Yoga. Practicing Re-membrance reawakens the "heart intelligence", plants the "heart seed" into fertile ground so that it can sprout a life that blooms a fragrance of praise. It brings to light, the golden threads that beckon us to our potential, so we can step forth both boldly, and in complete Trust of the Divine plan. It's a practice that uses the heart to reconnect the threads woven between the soul and the mind. I see it as a practice of light weaving, creating a cloth of reality that has all the points of connection in it, no longer severed by forgetting who we truly are, but reinforced by those light bearers who have come before us; and by this practice, are alive within us.

Bhakti Yoga is a treasure hunt of the Heart.

The Yoga of Re-membrance, is a practice of keeping the mind on an object which is an embodiment of transcendental consciousness. Transcendental, being that the person, object, or symbol has transcended the mundane, 3D, level of awareness, and is connected to a body of wisdom, a bigger picture, through a deepening of their evolution.

The act of remembering the name of the Divine, the act of remembering the Gurus in stories, creates a golden thread through time and space. It is this golden thread that, through remembrance, attunes your mind to calibrate to the frequency of the Guru Tattwa, the element of Light. When you Re-member, when you hear the stories of the enlightened ones, the ones who embody that frequency of light we call the Guru Tattwa, then your heart and mind align. A deep resonance is experienced and a remembering of your own soul aligning with its Indigenous Soul[1], the Self before all the crustaceans of ignorance has solidified and formed a new "reality", occurs. This resonance of Remembrance breaks through the shell of dormant potential into a visceral, living frequency from which to move through this life on Earth.

---

[1] Indigenous Soul - Term credited to Martin Prechtel, to describe the quality of being a part of Nature that is in humans, plants, and animals that exists as their most original and natural reality before the advent of big civilization; not specific to tribes or groups of people.

For life is a series of events and experiences that are forever trying to encourage us to walk the path of Love, by having us continually stumble into our self constructed walls of suffering and pain. And by choosing Love, we choose Grace.

There are some key definitions that help frame the perspective from which they are shared.

Discover and Remember:

Two words in the English language that, to me, epitomize the reason for living.

Dis-cover: To remove the coverings that hide that which is really there. The coverings, in yoga are called *maya*, being the dream, or the veil. When we identify with the Maya as being Truth we are in the experience called *avidya*; to not see clearly.

Re-member: to assemble pieces, members, that make up a wholeness, for whole is who we are.

To Re-member is not just a cognitive recalling of a memory that you allow the mind to ponder. It is a deep seeking in the silence of the Soul. Similarly, when you walk out of the room and you can't remember what you got up to get or do, you have to stand there and listen, search, try and recall the thread that employed action, often walking back to the place where you decided to act, hoping it will trigger the thread of memory. Re-membrance is the same practice, but on a soul level; searching for the thread that will reconnect you with the totality of your being, and activate a direct experience of living from the place of awareness of being completely interconnected with all beings.

We are able to practice this on different levels, working the muscles of perception from the mundane to the spiritual. Each level has its own importance, no level can be ignored on the path.

To step onto the path of Re-membrance, we must humbly admit that we have forgotten.

That there is nothing separate from us, nothing that we must acquire, or learn, but in fact it is a peeling away, a letting go of all that holds us in the illusion of separateness from that which is, and has always been there. A remembrance for what is, has been, and always will be; the completeness of who we are. In the ignorance of our identification with the human experience, we have clothed ourselves in beliefs and assumptions, labels and judgments, believing that we are building, creating who we are, instead of dissolving who we are not, until the humbling experience of being part of Creation Herself, The Divine Mother or Devi is presented to us.

Perspective and Perception:

These words create an orientation as to how we relate to an event and how we use this event to give meaning our lives.

Perspective: Is the container in which the ego cultivates and nourishes the story that is "I". It is the lower mind's declaration that what it sees is the Truth, rather than an acknowledgment of reality. Our perspective is the narrative that emboldens the ego's understanding, to believe that the way it sees and experiences a situation is the only be-all-and-end-all and thus is pushed onto others to agree. It is often the foundation for an argument or conflict.

The antidote being Humility - the magic frequency that expands the tight knot of a righteous perspective into an expanded experience of perception.

Perception: If perspective was the functioning of the lower mind or ego, then perception is the orientation of the higher mind, heart intelligence or the Soul. It can encompass and hold space for the reality of perspective, yet it is not limited to only that which the ego can "identify" with. It can empathize, loosen its grip on "the story" long enough to start to see patterns and weavings of cause and effect. It has space in it for the unseen, the indefinable, for that which lies just beyond the senses. It softens judgment to understanding. It reorients you to realizing that...

You are living in this world, but you are not of this world.

The way we orient the perception of our lives and why we are here on this Earth has the potential to hold our perspective as the orientation point of which we currently stand and what we are here to learn, without it being a definition of who or what we are. There's room for magic to rush in and show us another way.
As a Human race, we are at the brink of an opportunity to evolve faster and farther than we ever have before as the darkness or ignorance embodied during the Kali Yuga[2] gives birth to an intense light that is there for the basking. It is an opportunity for each of us to decide where our reality will lie, which paradigm of consciousness we will seat ourselves in. Our life is the opportunity to fully experience, and appreciate the dualism of the light and dark, which we can see so clearly in our relationship with the Divine through Mother Earth. This opportunity to transcend this

---

[2] Kali Yuga: the lastof the four stages (or ages or Yugas) the world goes through as part of a 'cycle of Yugas'. It is one of discord and strife as human civilization is thought to degenerate spiritually being referred to as the Dark Age because in it people are as far away as possible from God.

perspective of dualism is one of the gifts of this human experience on earth. Only when we live from the perspective that we are separate from others, and from the Earth do we dare pillage or take more than what is sustainable for the overall health of the Whole. When we perceive our interconnectedness with All we no longer seek to hold power over the "other"; instead we shift into genuine gratitude for all the intricate pieces that are playing their role in our perceived reality.

Perspective and Perception become rungs on a ladder of consciousness. We always stand at our perspective, always reaching out for that which we perceive. Once we full integrate, understand and embody that which we perceive, our handhold becomes our new foothold and we stand at a new level of perspective, allowing us to reach further to a new level of perception.

The teachings, processes or paths on how to do this, travelling from perspective or mundane mind to perception or spiritual mind, has been held by many different lineages, or schools of philosophy in many different parts of the world at different times, including the ones that have fully influenced my life, Vedanta, Tantra and Yoga. The teachings of these paths, are medicine for the Soul and are not limited, nor owned, by one race or another. The Divine Mother, Great Spirit, Parusha, Prakriti, Wancatonka, The Holy in Nature or whatever your particular culture calls the force of the Divine behind this dream we call life, is there for all to Remember and embody. However, there have been cultures that have been more successful in holding these "Truths" tangible and more pure than others. The Indians in the Himalayas have kept intact the philosophies of Tantra, Vedanta and the techniques of Yoga throughout the ages. The Native Americans have kept intact their ability and insights of the Great Spirit. South America has their versions through the shamans, Russian culture has their thread of Remembrance of the Vedic culture as can be seen though the recent books of Anastasia. These philosophies are not of a skin colour, or a geographical appropriation, and although there are many paths, they are, and will always be, for the Remembrance of the Soul. These philosophies, or "old ways", are important for ALL who genuinely seek, and for those who are willing to step into right action and alignment to be able to receive the teachings. Now, please note that I'm not talking about different religions holding the Truth, I'm talking about cultures that acknowledge Spirit, The Divine, whatever you want to call it, in their day to day life. I'm talking about cultures that embody a paradigm of *perception* that is inclusive, not exclusive, and has room for whichever face of God you wish to identify with, without it holding power over anyone else's belief or experience. Polytheism, not Mono-theism.

The reality is, each of these cultures have had to bring the teachings underground to keep them as pristine as possible, untainted by greed and beyond the blinding dualism and ignorance that permeates the Kali Yuga.

Anytime we are fully identified with the us and them, the black or white, cop or crook, Democrat or Republican we are functioning from a 3D perspective. The key word here is "identified". It's not that we don't experience this duality, it's when we believe in the us and them on a mental and emotional level, our ability to see, or our perception of what really is at play, is limited. We are rendered unable to recognize the perfection in the cycles of the leela, or play of the Divine, that is this life.

Our experience in this lifetime is, at the moment, about ninety to one hundred years max, yet the cycles of the Earth, and the cycles of states of consciousness or Yugas are into the hundreds of thousands. We, our Souls, ask to come and be a part of a collective consciousness, to allow our individual mind frequency to hold space and amplify as much light as we can for the time we are here, but in reality, we are but a minuscule blip on the radar of the Divine. This is not to minimize the importance or the gift of our opportunities as humans, for we sit in the beauty of the macro and the micro - as above, so below. What we each individually do is extremely important in the amount of light and frequency we are able to embody and utilize on Earth. And yet, it is God's gift to us that we use the present, this moment, right here, to breathe in gratitude, and breathe out all the layers of "I" that no longer serves us so it can be realigned to its rightful place in the Universe. Humans are part of God's opportunity to forget itself, so God too, can Re-member. It is a collective shift in our overall perception of life itself to truly Re-member as we are not individual, rather a part of the whole.

Frequency of Attunement:

Frequency of attunement: Refers to a vibration of light or sound that can be calibrated to open up different perceptions of understanding and new perspectives on reality.

Different levels of perception Re-member in different ways. For the mundane or gross, 3rd Dimensional level of perception it's about stimulating remembrance though action, e.g., a photo, stories, the great texts, fables, verbal storytelling of the ancestors, chanting mantras or yoga ecology practices that utilize our connection with nature as the portal to the forgotten. On the mundane level of the mind these are actions that we do, and we get comfort, enjoyment, and teachings from them.

In yoga, one of the five Niyamas, or personal observances, is called Swadhyaya. This usually is translated as "self-study" or "one's own reading" and is often further expressed as taking time to read the Vedic texts e.g., the Bhagavad Gita. It is taught as the effort of studying and analyzing oneself for development and transformation. There can be a third take on "Swadhyaya" in that Swadhyaya is immersing oneself in the stories, studies and teachings of the great Vedic works, not to learn them, but to expose oneself to the transmissions, the frequencies of light, that they imbibe. This connects to frequencies of Remembrance to the subtle mind and is experienced as deep contemplative listening that rekindles that heart into a knowing that is beyond doubt.

The immersion of Swadhyaya in this way, gives one a direct experience of these frequencies to be able to attune yourself, your own resonance, to theirs, thus embodying and realigning at a core level the wisdom and teachings of these texts to which their frequency will naturally start to be absorbed and expressed by you.

This process changes the point of frequency beyond the mind. Allowing a shift to naturally filter down though the sheaths of perception or what we call in Yoga, the Koshas, rather than physically analyzing words to try and push consciousness further up the chain of awareness by brute mental force.

This completely resonates with me - pardon the pun - in the practice of Re-membrance. These texts have multiple layers of teachings and symbology accessible to offering transformation or solace at different parts of the mind. Yet, they are also texts, nay - stories, that are alive, they are a song of light weaving, a reality beyond, overcoming conflict, beyond multiple arms and blue skin. They are a transmission of potential, a pathway to Re-membering the totality of which we are a part of, from which we stem from.

So at a mundane level we have the actions, the reading, the chanting, but with the aspiration and awareness that what we are truly opening to is not a intellectual recounting or understanding, but by reading the books, listening to the stories, from a yogic perspective, such as the *Ramacharitamanas*, or chanting the *Sundari Lahara* we are in fact humbly opening ourselves to the unknown, the forgotten. For unless we use a tool, regardless of which sense it comes through, a photo, a chant, a book or practice of nature connection, we are only limiting ourselves to remember that which the ego's limited perspective will acknowledge. Your ego can remember the forgotten, about as well as it can think its way into unthinking.

The process of Re-membrance is not an intellectual regurgitation of details, but an opening to a feeling, a frequency that the person or event embodies - even if they are not longer in body.

Using Remembrance in this way is opening the perceptional gating of the mind into a different state of consciousness. It is bringing Heart intelligence to the forefront, through feeling, into every moment, an injection of light and heart overpowering the relentless hold of the intellect on reality. Just for one moment, you experience a feeling as a primary sensorial indicator of soul meeting world, rather than mind meeting reality.

There is a difference between living in the past, and using the power of Remembrance to expand the gating of consciousness. Living in the past, be the memories positive or negative, hold the consciousness in the shadows of emotion, fear, grief, attachment, shame, and guilt. Even positive memories, when reminiscing will hold a thin casing of sadness, of longing, of grief in the awareness that the time is gone and cannot be brought back.

However, when the mind returns to remembering people, places or events that are of a spiritual nature, the frequency of these memories actually pries open the consciousness into pools of trust, surrender, and contentment, for we realize that the frequencies we are remembering do not belong in the past, but fragments of multidimensional light that are as alive in this present moment as any other. By Re-membering the Light (bearers) one injects the frequency of the Guru Tattwa into their field of consciousness, thus making it a very powerful tool for recalibration throughout the day.

In some of the stories in this book, the light cracks through my awareness of reality like a fine sliver of glass just under the skin; you can't see it, but you can't *not* feel it either. In other stories, the light blows my sense of reality up, making the possibility of returning to the old level of awareness unfathomable. But in each of these stories is a pivotal moment of Grace — a moment beyond my conscious control that, for me, holds the teachings of yoga in a this-life-this-moment way, and through these, the potential of a delicious Re-membering of the nature of my Indigenous Soul.

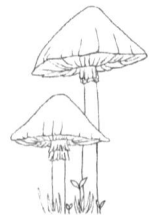

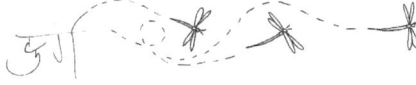

ONE

- Ma Durga Jai Ho

Stepping onto the Path of Bhakti Yoga and wading into the ocean of Re-membrance, as a practice of attunement, is most of the time, for me, a playful dance between the discipline of a practice or Sadhana and Surrender, being open to what comes without control or expectation. Between imagination, letting the heart guide through the feeling sense, and discernment, the thinking that gauges right action, after all this information is gathered, seeks to be digested into a place that is kind and safe within your inner and outer reality.

Using Sadhana to create a personal and customized vocabulary with the Divine through Nature is a wonderfully liberating experience that really allows you to *feel* a direct link in communication without having to go through a third party or authority. To be able to hear the song of the Divine Spirit, the practice of Mantra, hands down, is my favourite way to do this. Mantra is a practice of using the Sanskrit language to stimulate, absorb and align specific frequencies within our consciousness. Mantra sets the frequency that allows an experience to unfold into our reality. It comes from the two root words of Manas, meaning the mind, and Trayati, meaning to expand or liberate. So Mantra is the practice of liberating the mind from its identified bindings to experience expanded states of consciousness.

I like the Sadhana of Mantra to guide me towards the symbolism required to fulfill my intention at the time. It might lead me to a specific tree, or to a spot where I interact with a specific animal or bird. I like the heart to lead the seeking of symbolism through totems, witnessing my own experience and, most importantly, the *feeling* behind the interaction. Then, after I have been through this personal volley between focusing on the symbol or totem and checking in with my heart sense, or the feelings that arise with that focus, Then I seek out the 'medicine' or symbology of this further through books and other analytical references. I bounce between this outer, analytical thinking, body of information, and inner, analogical tracking, until a reality I can digest and integrate forms - one that I can feel nourishing my soul. It is important to be willing to create your own communication and experience with the totem or symbol before trying to impose someone else's definition upon your experience. Consciously listen to both the heart and the mind as two valid bodies of information that give multidimensionality to the point of focus. This in and of itself becomes the foundation of sovereignty and a life of direct connection with the Divine.

I'm often asked if I will translate the Mantras we are learning into English. People want to "know" the "words" they are "singing" to intellectually decide if they "believe" it or not. While theoretically you can translate the Sanskrit into English words it would be like trying to write a word for each note of Beethoven's Moonlight Sonata to decide if you liked the piece or not. Music and Mantra are languages of the Soul, not the intellect. You feel them, you explore them internally, you don't rationalize them, you soak them in and let their notes and sounds recalibrate your perspective on reality.

Salvatore, a beloved mentor, friend and soul brother of mine, (who also graciously wrote the foreword of this offering) once shared a story with me that made an impact on my perception of the vast complexities of the Sanskrit language, Mantras, and how the nuances of the language we use, in fact, creates that reality we perceive.

One evening in the late fall of 1982, Pandit Usharbudh Arya *(the late Swami Veda Bhāratī) took me to an Indian dance recital at the University of Minnesota. Afterward, we went out for ice cream and I took the moment to ask questions that had been on my mind for some time.*

The fact that Sanskṛit was his native language intrigued me in several ways and led to my first question, "Pandiji, is there anyone in the world you can actually talk to with full ease and comprehension?"

He replied, "At any point in time, three thousand to five thousand Indians list Sanskṛit as their cradle language (14,000 in 2015, ed). So, yes, there are people I can talk with. However, the form of Sanskṛit I grew up speaking is quite specialized and I have only my sister for absolutely fluent conversations."

This struck me as necessarily having a quality of deep solitude, if not loneliness, and led to the next question, "What is it like for you to speak English?"

His expression changed to what I interpreted as sadness. He gently placed a hand on my forearm and said, "I don't want you to feel badly, but for me speaking English is like you talking 'baby talk.' There is so much from my culture and tradition I would love to share with you, but simply cannot. We have concepts in Sanskṛit that have no equivalents in English. Without the concepts, there can be no descriptive vocabulary. In fact, the English grammar is too limited as well. Entire libraries in India cannot be translated." He paused for a moment and then brightened up. "However," he enthused, "with the advent of the Theory of Relativity, quantum mechanics, and particle physics, the West is on a path of convergence. If the West continues at its present rate, in its present direction, of scientific discovery, these books should translatable in one to two hundred years."

We sat in silence. I have to admit that I was less than overjoyed by his prediction, but it propelled me into a thought-

direction that has occupied a significant portion of my life investigation ever since. As I experienced the conversation, Arya was implying that there were thoughts that were unthinkable in English. BIG thoughts! My experience living on Native American reservations during my university years had made me quite aware that different people could experience and interpret the same phenomena in dramatically different ways. However, the idea that entire ranges of reality might be outside a cultural scope of perception had never occurred to me. [3]

Sanskrit, in my experience, being that I am not an intellectual scholar of the language, is one of transmission. Aligning my mundane mind with the words of light is like making a deposit into an account at a bank. Each Mantra said is a deposit into an account that dates back thousands of years. Each repetition by each soul has been deposited into this account creating a force field of light that is beyond space and time. Each time we chant something like the Maha Mantra - Hari Krishna Hari Krishna, Krishna Krishna, Hari Hari... we are simultaneously offering our deposit, and receiving a pure, amplified stream of light from the account into our energy bodies. Each Mantra has its own account or bubble of light, and when used with sincerity can be an incredible tool to help navigate our mundane reality by bathing it in a spiritually illuminated perspective. This is how we change our dimensional paradigm. Not by hiding in caves, or running away from our worldly commitments, but by keeping this door open in a part of our minds as we move through our daily actions.

In "The Great Mission", a book about the life and start of Rabbi Yisrael Baal Shem Tov is a wonderful quote linked into a Jewish/Hebrew perspective of the same teaching. It reads:

---

[3] Taken from the essay "Language, Thought, and Reality" from the Introduction to The Yoga-Sutra Sanskrit-English Dictionary.

"Man is constantly overwhelmed by daily frustrations. While trying to earn a livelihood and provide for his family, man encounters many difficulties along the way. These frustrations can be compared to the great Deluge, a flood of problems that threaten to drown our spiritual ambitions. What is the solution to this dilemma? '[G-d said to Noah:] Enter the ark, you and your household'" (Genesis 7:1)

Playing on the Hebrew word teiva - which can mean either "ark" or "word" - the Baal Shem Tov interpreted this verse to underscore the unique quality of Torah and Prayer. "Enter the tieva," he explained. "Come into the sacred words of the Torah and prayer, thereby forming a protective barrier against the menacing waters of our physical world."

From a Yogic perspective, this is completely aligned with the teaching that through Mantra, sacred words that are beyond mere translation, you are able to take shelter, ark/word, from the deluge of water, the emotional identification of unconscious flowing impressions into your conscious reality. In other words, to take a safe place in navigating the turbulent waters of reality, take shelter in the Name.

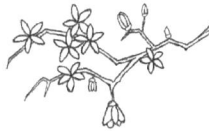

It was this way of working, through the Sadhana of the well known Gayatri Mantra, that created a deeply foundational experience for me in 2006 when I was in Costa Rica on a Yoga Retreat with my teacher Anandashakti.

We had spent a week engaged in multiple classes and Sadhanas, as well as enjoying the local sights and opportunities. Sweet and sticky fried plantain and freshly pureed mango juice for breakfasts, sitting on sun warmed rocks at sacred waterfalls for lunch. I fell in love with the way the humidity there envelops your soul into a cradling of whispered sonnets. How the forest pulses at a beat you have no choice but to dance to. It's a celebration of life, interconnectedness, all living beings as part of a self generating symphony and your presence at the party is a *fait accompli.*

On the last evening we all sat beside the swimming pool, basking in the light of the full moon from both above and from the moon's reflection off the water. Not a single beam was wasted, like the English holding up a sheet of tin under their chins on a rare English sunny day, we were determined to absorb as much luna light before returning to the reality of city life the next day.

The prescribed Sadhana for the evening was of course the Gayatri Mantra, each syllable a drop of elixir on the tongue, but alas for me, that particular night Her medicine was bitter. Like a nebulizer, mantra electrifies and purifies the atmosphere, simultaneously stimulating the absorption and emission of light. But where there is light on this earthly plain, there is darkness. And if the mind is hiding an infection in the shadows, Mantra will bring it directly to the surface for examination and the opportunity to heal. My mental defenses on this particular evening were no match for the collective force of light created by the group. The drone of voices dredged forth in me layers of resistance, then irritability and like a mosquito that won't land when you're trying to sleep, my thoughts circled, perseverating on my current relationship, an illusive, yet suffocating, push-me-pull-you. Stoically, I sat though the chanting and the visualizations that were offered but was relieved when it was over and we were able to retire for the evening.

The last instructions given to us were to use the energy of the Mantra to ask the Divine Mother to show herself to us in a dream that night. To allow us to experience her form in whatever way was in our most high. Of course, I followed the suggestion and set the intention but gratefully fell fast into, for the most part, a dreamless sleep. To my surprise, as I'm not one to often remember my dreams, sometime in the night, my one and only memorable dream was that the Divine Mother came to me as a huge Dragonfly. The dream itself was underwhelming. There was no life changing wisdom that was imparted. Not that I could remember anyway. There was no 'scene' or play out of a story. It was simple and brief. A single image of remembrance - a huge Dragonfly before me announcing Herself as the Divine Mother. I was reluctant to express the next morning that She had shown Herself to me as a really large insect, so apart from letting my teacher know I kept it to myself.

Like all good quality seeds, my Ma as a dragonfly, lay dormant in my heart waiting for the right conditions to take root and sprout. Sometimes showing up in random places, perhaps so I would not forget all together, here and there in photos or at the pond briefly saying "hello", infusing my day with the kind of childlike joy. That was, until one day she decided to sprout and take her rooted place as a beacon for my life to follow on the 14th August 2009, my wedding day.

The blessed day of Krishna Janmashtami was chosen for us by a Swami to be the day of our wedding as it was the day that the God of love, Krishna, was born. This particular year it landed on a Friday, ruled by the Goddess of love Herself - Venus. It was important to us that the main ceremony be centered around a Vedic Havan, conducted by the same teacher I had gone to Costa Rica with Anandashakti. There we gathered in traditional western wedding attire, in an English country garden in Woodstock Connecticut, but instead of standing in front of a minister, we were seated at the cardinal directions around a fire. Warm sun illuminated each individual leaf on the surrounding trees, each one waving hello as we set up and prepared. There was a slight breeze, only enough for fairies to dance upon, stimulating an olfactory meal of fresh flowers, incense, sandalwood and rose. We were surrounded by 21 family members and friends, and for most, this was their first experience of such a ceremony. I'll never forget my father-in-law, as sandalwood oil was delicately dotted between his eye brows, exclaiming that until that moment he was unaware that he had a third eye! The Bija Mantras, or seed sounds in Sanskrit, were easy to pronounce, and everyone chanted with full heart, calling out and beckoning the Divine beings to bless our souls together in a life of marriage.

After the ceremony, when all the traditional and not so traditional commemorative photos had been taken, only my teacher, Anandashakti, my new husband, Paramjyoti, our good friend and wedding photographer Pete and myself were left outside in the garden. Relieved that everything had gone very well, me, my eight and a half month pregnant belly and my swollen feet found a place to rest a moment on an old, rough concrete bench. As I sat amidst the quaint flowering plants, Narayana, the being temporarily residing inside me, thought we were already in the dancing part of the evening and was wriggling and kicking up a storm. With one hand on my belly trying to sooth my mini Michael Jackson, I looked over towards my teacher who was looking up with a cross between delight and astonishment across her face. "Look!" she said pointing to the space above our heads. As equal part that my eyes looked up, my jaw dropped. To our amazement, there were thousands, and I mean thousands, of Dragonflies circling above us in a tornado of wings.

"Ma Durga Jai Ho!"

She had come, she had heeded our call in the Havan, to dance on the birthday of Love and make an appearance at our wedding showering on us her abundance of blessings.

From that day, I committed to myself that any Odonata, the order to which both Dragonflies and Damselflies belong, would be a direct communication to me from ma Durga. The experience in

Costa Rica with Ma Dragonfly had been my first toe towards diving in to the Ocean of Remembrance. From this seed, the muscle of listening, trusting, dreaming and surrendering all started to be stimulated into a framework for a new reality. My wedding solidified it into an undeniable compass to navigate my life on the path of Bhakti Yoga and Remembrance. At first it was like working a muscle that had long ago atrophied, and yet, since then, I have no idea how I functioned without it.

Me, sitting on the bench on our wedding day, looking at Ma Dragonfly shower her blessings on us.

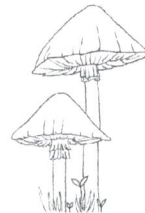

Now, every time I see a Dragonfly, either in nature or just an image, the Archetypal frequency of the Divine mother is stimulated inside of me, often disrupting my mental flow just long enough for me to check in with my heart and my breath and become present with what she is showing me in this moment. Upon seeing one I always exclaim "Ma Durga Jai Ho!" as a joyful wink of acknowledgement to the Divine that I am being watched, guided and supported every step of the way.

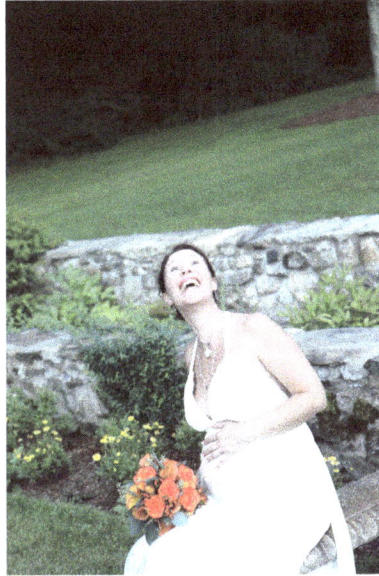

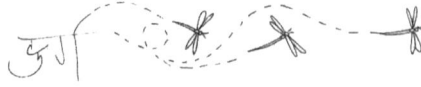

TWO

- Tabula Rasa.

In order to open to Re-membrance, we must first acknowledge that maybe, we have forgotten. That maybe somewhere along the way, over many lifetimes even, we have stepped away from embodying our place in the complete interconnectedness of Nature, and have compartmentalized, fractured our souls in the name of *civilization*. Alas, life is the leela[4] of the Gods. A play so grand that you forget you are acting. Embodying our parts so well as to be fully i-dentified in the experience of forgetting, so we have the joy of remembering; to fall down, so we have the opportunity to rise; to die, over and over so we can once again experience the miracle of birth. Again and again we forget our true Nature, so we can experience our way into Remembering. The journey of this we know as Evolution. Really, the complete encompassing, omnipotent, omnipresent consciousness that I call God, The Holy in Nature, or Great Spirit, to which our soul is an aspect, is itself experiencing itself, Poornamadah[5]. The reality of dualism is a slight of God's hand, so that in our ignorance - a distracted state of forgetfulness, we are able to Re-member - experience the truth of Atmabhav or the Attitude of Oneness. The facets (as in individual face) of a diamond would swear the outlook to be completely different, that 'their' perspective was important/unique, and it is, but no more important or unique than the face-t next to it. In fact, without the face-t next to it, its

---

[4]Leela: the play

[5] Poornamadah: The teaching that everything is an experience of the same whole that can never have anything added to it, nor taken away.

perspective would not be what it is, they are completely interdependent, completely connected aspects of a whole who's outlook on the "outside" world is different. And while the facet itself holds a perspective, its very mass or substance that it is made from is indefinable and completely integrated into the diamond itself. Each one of us, each bird, each dog, each tree, are holding our face-t in the perfection of a luminous diamond.

We are all part of a great song, one note in a symphony. To believe we are the conductor is foolish and audacious. To instead embrace the few notes we have the privilege to play, and offer them as a sweet, sincere act of beauty that bubbles up from our childlike exuberance is really what we need to focus our life-force energy on.

Each stage of our evolutionary perspective has a philosophy, tools and wisdom to keep it stepping further forward, to help it remember the totality of ONE. Different stages can therefore, sometimes, seem contradictory in their teachings. Consider how you might point out the seed of a flower lying on the ground. The person then learns that seeds are found on the ground in a certain colour and texture. And then at another time you see the inside of a blossom of a flower, and are told that this is the seed of the same flower. As we expand our understanding of the life cycle and patterns of consciousness and Nature we are able to hold certain contradictions with the expanded nuances of awareness.

But how do you grasp the concept of Atmabhava, the attitude of ONEness, or SubEk - All one, when we are constantly experiencing our lives as a seemingly series of isolated events colliding with each other to create our reality? Thunder and Lightening. We experience them as different things, for different senses read them in different places in space and time. Yet, they are two words for the same phenomenon. Thunder and lightening are not two different phenomenons, they do not exist separately, it is because of the maya or illusion of time and space, and our languaging that we consider them to be two different things. It's the same of the concept of "you" and "me", or "humans" and the "earth". Just because we label and experience them in a time space continuum as being separate, does not make that reality the Truth.

As we start to experience a softening around our containers of *reality*, a pause in our hard-edged language of labels and identification, a feathering of what we *know* to be time, space, reality, and truth, we start to open to experiences beyond the duality of what our senses tell us. We start to receive deep impulses, sparks of Remembrance that we cannot rationally explain. Impulses that are birthed from a deep place of softness within us, that compel us to action in what the outside world likes to label as "an episode", but what the soul experiences as a deep re-collection, an experience of past, present and future to finally collide into this moment of deep listening, of deep Remembrance.

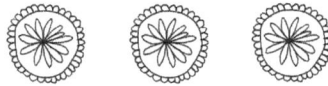

So imagine this. It's 2006 and here I am, a twenty-six year old, white woman. I'm not overly polished, a little hard headed, skeptical, impulsive, raw, yet honest and clearly ready for change. Still in that mid twenties state of searching for something on the outside of myself, I've moved from Toronto to Vancouver to be a "yoga teacher" having just finished my 650 Hour Teacher training the year before. I've taken a somewhat spontaneous trip to India at the behooving of a Swami I had met only a couple of times and I am, for the first time in my life, genuinely aware of how much of a mess I am, with a sprinkling of admittance that I don't know what I'm doing, but I'm going to do it with gusto. Being a Gemini with Libra and Pisces in the mix, composed of air and water, just like a Dragonfly, I move quickly when I put my mind to it, and yet, a part of me is home in the deep waters of emotion. I have a sensitive underbelly that I've learnt to keep hidden behind my fire.

Kolkata; like me, it too is a city of extremes. Parts of it are manicured to the placement of a blade of grass and parts are the dirtiest embodiment of filth you can imagine. It has money paving the courtyards of five star hotels and slums that humble the hardest layers of a fearful entitled heart. And here I am, sitting somewhere in between in a modest hotel restaurant, eating a breakfast that is a little too spicy for my digestive system first thing in the morning, nervously anticipating my first trip to an bonafide Ashram with a real "enlightened Master", whatever that means. But surely by having gone there, I too will have more credibility in my yoga teaching and maybe I will be celebrated for 'just how far I have come'.

Mid mouthful of my turmeric infused meal, a deep compulsion smacks me on the side of the head - I need to shave my head, right now, in this moment. Now, I could argue that it was a deep calling of the Soul, a remembering of perhaps lifetimes gone by that had me almost spit out my food and announce this necessity to the man sitting next to me. I could convince you that somewhere in me there was a knowing that there was life before that morning and there would be life after, but that in that moment it was a beginning, a clean slate, a Tabula Rasa and I needed an action to acknowledge that. It could also be said that I wanted to, as usual, fit in and be liked while simultaneously setting myself apart from the ordinary folk with the latest hair-do,

or hair-don't as the case maybe.

Regardless which one holds the most truth, there is a humbling little bit of reality in all of them. Without skipping a beat, the man sitting next to me, instantly got up, and walked towards the door, with a sparkle in his eye, challenging me to walk the walk, he casually replied "ok well let's do it then".

Walking out of the hotel and onto the street, decomposing particles of scent assaulted my skin like a warm, damp hug of decay. Stepping into the hustle and bustle of Kolkata's morning oblations, my new friend walked straight up to a slight Muslim man who despite working on the side of the pavement in Kolkata as a barber appeared to be remarkably clean. It was communicated between the two men that on account of him, the barber, being Muslim, he was reluctant to shave a woman's head and even more opposed to shaving a western woman's head. However, the gleaming appearance of a 50 rupee note first thing in the morning soon had him whistling a different tune. He gestured me to have a seat upon his barbering throne, an upturned wooden box, and through grunts and bobbing implied he wanted me to flip my hair over and assume the position of my head almost between my knees. After blessing me with freezing cold Kolkata bacteria filled water upon my head, he proceeded to reconcile a tango between his straight razor and my manicured mahogany locks. Ten minutes later, my heart having been lulled with the distracting rhythm of splash splash, mumble mumble, adjust head, scrap, he suddenly stops. Too terrified to open my eyes, as though I would be able to see my newly born reflection in his eyes, I waited for him to say something, but the clang of the razor hitting a metal bowl was all that was communicated the dance was over and at last I peeked at my new reality. The barber was off chatting to friends and my breakfast buddy was patiently waiting for me to emerge. My elbow length locks were crouched in the Kolkata gutter like a kitten being surrounded by a pack of wolves. Motionless, clearly the odd one out and resigned to its fate.

Back in my hotel room, having beckoned a cheerful "see ya in a few" to my breakfast buddy I ushered myself into the bathroom where time bent and fractured within its tiled walls. My breath was suspended indefinitely, as my heart thundered at warp speed. I was somewhat grateful there was a toilet standing by.

Then slowly, very, very slowly, I looked in the mirror.

I stood there, paralyzed between curious and terrified. I simultaneously, greeted the alien before me, and yet, reflected in its eyes; it was as though I was truly meeting my-Self for the very first time. Clean, clear, no memory of the past, raw, uncomplicated, present, birthed. I could see myself without distraction, the way I needed to, to step forth in this experience without hiding behind anything. Tears streaked the slightly reddened face, but in my eyes, a bright blue azure being was staring at me with recognition and inquisitiveness. Who are you?

After completing my formal introductions to this new reflection, I haphazardly wrapped my head in a scarf, pulled up my big girl pants, put on my 'no big deal' face and went and got on a train to the Ashram.

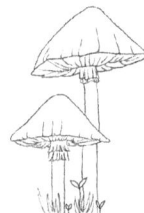

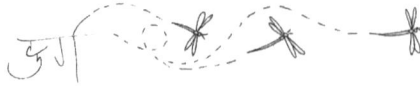

THREE

- Walking The Walk

The transition from mundane awareness to the transitional bridge of waking up can be clunky. I've never found it to be a straight line, it's more like a fox trot. I have found it to be, at times, painful, confusing, and feeling a little like I'm hitting the evolutional snooze button, all the while knowing full well that I'm alive to learn and evolve as a soul, by having this human experience. Sometimes it's like I almost commit to awakening to the new day and then collapse back into the engulfing void of blissful sleep, ignorance and potato chips. It's here, if we are lucky, that Grace takes the form of that life changing teacher. The form of a bitter pill that nevertheless makes you healthier.

We all experience Grace. Flashes of light that for a brief moment illuminate a new way of Being, beaconing us to embrace the present opportunity and let go of the old ways of doing things that hold us in suffering. The mundane calls it luck, the yogis call it Grace or blessings, the Masters call it Love of and unto itself. Grace is guidance and opportunities gifted by the Divine. A tipping point moment that is infused with a new frequency long enough that you can *experience* a new reality, shifting a pattern forever. Not to say that you won't experience the aftershocks of those patterns. The aftershocks are like a spiral of experience. They keep coming back, but in slightly nuanced ways. They are the Divine's way of saying, "Are you sure you get the lesson? Are you really sure?" And yet the first time you change direction from a pattern so ingrained in your psyche that you didn't realize there was another way of being, is nothing short of a miracle manifested.

However, like any skill, to recognize Grace's song in the hustle and bustle of the mind is a dance with trial and error. To humble yourself to its fullest potential is a process, to harness its momentum takes considerable awareness. To practice Remembrance towards it, to let its memory spark the light in the heart — this is the Magic. So while Grace is offered to every soul, not every soul can recognize its face and harness the potential. You must prepare.

Grace is the song of Divine Will, that pushes and nudges you into your highest. When you learn to recognize its tune it gives you comfort and courage to continue in that dance. When you don't recognize its song, it passes by you like music playing from a passing car. A glimpse of recognizing the tune, but no real grasp of the lyrics and thus its message.

Grace, Guru and God are the same light that dispels the darkness. I no longer recognize them as being separate experiences. The darkness being the ignorant beliefs that hold you in the mental patterning of suffering. For example, the dualistic identification of the archetypal patterns or stories we tell of our realities from the perspective of such as victim/perpetrator, co-dependant/caretaker or aloof/interrogator. To dispel these beliefs, to change this pattern, you have to face them and that includes taking responsibility for your part in them. - *often the trickiest part.* They have to play out in your reality and face the deep rut in the psyche that employs you to do the same response over and over, sometimes for lifetimes, and instead, you have to consciously choose a different response. In turn, opening to a reality you, until then, didn't even realize existed, sending out new frequency ripples into the cosmos.

There is no better place to face the manifestation of your own ignorance than an Ashram. The word Ashram means "place of work". That is not to say it's a manual labour camp, albeit that is sometimes what it looks like from the outside, but rather a place where great work on the internal plane takes place. It is a scrubbing station for the ego, to dispel ignorance so that your inner light can shine. And boy does it work...

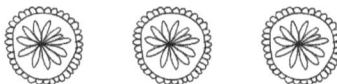

* * *

This was mirrored to me a few weeks after arriving for my first stay in the Ashram. Having taken a tour of the surrounding communities, of mud huts and humble means, we were walking back to the main compound along the long, dusty red snake of a road that warms its blood all day basking in the sun. At one point it was pointed out to a small group of us that the Master, this "Sri Swamiji" lived in that building over there. Looking in the distance of two or three different buildings I asked for clarification as to if it was the one with a satellite or the one without. This, I was to find out later, was a trigger of great magnitude for our Swami guide.

The next morning I was pulled out of our morning class by this particular Swami and ripped to pieces exclaiming that he had received multiple complaints about me since my arrival at the Ashram. Not stating who had the problem with me, or exactly what I had done, it was expressed that my rude statement of judgment as to if a Master should be allowed a satellite or not, was not my concern, and my irreverence was a direct reflection on him, as he was the one that had brought me to the Ashram in the first place. Genuinely confused as to how using the only obvious difference between two buildings as a descriptor somehow became an exclamation of judgment I tried to explain, to convince, to exonerate myself of wrong doing. This is how I had always gone about conflict. And as usual, nothing I said made an iota of difference to the situation. I had made a grave error and was officially outcast from his, the swami's, good books.

For as long as I could remember I had a pattern of "being accused of things" I didn't do, a pattern of things I had said being taken out of context, misunderstood - or miscommunicated. It had always devastated me to believe that someone I respected or loved would think ill of me.

But as grace would have it, it was this time, this irrational scolding that flipped a switch in me. It turned me a 180 and instead of needing my teacher to think well of me I went inside.

I remember thinking, 'Well, I know what I said, and I know what I meant by it, and I truly was not being malicious or disrespectful. Ignorant maybe, but not malicious. So, if I know what I said, and this "enlightened master", who I have not yet laid eyes on, who is reported to being omnipresent, omnipotent, and God intoxicated as everyone says, then He will know what I said and what I meant. And really, if I truly am in a place where people can truly evolve by the Grace of the frequencies of a Tapobhoomi[6] and a Paramahansa[7] as this "Sri Swamiji" is said to be, then this Sri Swamiji's opinion is the only one I need be concerned with. So, I no longer care what you think. I only care what He thinks.'

Grace often reveals its form as the courage it takes to seek out the light reflecting back in the eyes of habitual despair.

For the last week and a half of my Ashram stay I kept my distance from said Swami. I was kind and courteous but not vying for his attention or approval as I had been. Each time I felt that fear

---

[6] Tapobhoomi: From two words (1) Tapo : from tapas meaning austerities meaning - Purification at practical level - purification of body, kind, emotions and spirit ultimately leading to one pointedness. This one pointedness is the highest austerity demanding the highest level of attention, perpetually on one's inner being. Bhumi: Land, Place - In this respect - A place where Sadhana if internalizing one's attention is practiced. A place for performance of austerities.

[7] Paramahamsa: Param means Supreme or ultimate... and Hamsa means Swan... Paramahamsa means a Sadhak who has reached a stage where he can discriminate between Truth and Maya (illusion)

of being rejected I turned my stubborn mind to the solace that if I knew I hadn't done anything wrong, then "Sri Swamiji" would too. This gave me a new mental frequency, a new internal "story" or thread of thought to hold onto. In doing so, it shifted something inside me to a deeper level of strength and trust in something other than myself that was simultaneously intangible, and a frequency of such strength and envelopment, that it could not be ignored. When I look back now, this was my first conscious experience of active Faith and Surrender - a letting go of the power of appearances, and perception, and a shifting to a faith of a bigger picture, yet unseen but no less real, on a mundane level of awareness.

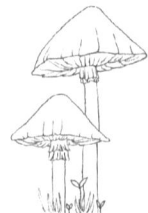

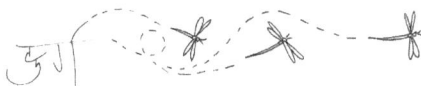

FOUR

- Meeting A Master

Jesus was, and is, a Guru. A being of light who had mastered the Re-membrance of his true self while being in a human experience. A being who taught the importance of Love, Compassion, Service, who embodied Christ consciousness and who set the example of living in this world, but not being *of* this world. He lived by example, gave inspiration to those who met him, and all those who cherish the Bible, those who aspire to live in a way that is inching closer to their fullest potential as He did. Gu-ru means dispeller of darkness. A Guru is a being so bright, that your shadow evaporates, albeit temporarily, just by being in their presence, by reading their words which hold transmission, or by Re-membering them.

Jesus was a remarkable soul who touched down on this earth to anchor a frequency of Love. Yet he was not and is not the only soul that has been able to achieve this embodiment of God intoxication. Anandamayi Ma, Neem Karoli Baba, Swami Śivananda, Rabbi Yisrael Baal Shem Tov, Amma, and Buddha to name just a few, as there are others out there, in the public eye and out of it, that are and have quietly embodied and emanated the frequency of pure Love on this Earth.

By Re-membering the en-lightened ones, we are actually collecting light towards us. For the frequency of the Guru Tattwa, the element of light, is not an external experience, but an internal one. We associate with beings that have embodied this frequency of expanded awareness, both through stories and in person, as a point of connection providing a chance to calibrate our own core frequency into a higher frequency of our innate Self. This can be a challenging concept for people who only look at what their eyes can see, and only feel what they can intellectualize. When we only "believe" what our personality or ego will justify, our soul has to sit quietly until our ego is in crisis, or exhausted, before it will start to open up to letting the soul take the helm of this human experience. How many people have to be terminally ill, before they start prioritizing qualities, that of which are intangible i.e. kindness, generosity, selflessness, over material quantities i.e. the car, the house, the vacation?

When speaking of the importance of engaging with an outer Guru, until the internal Guru can be attuned to, Anandamayi Ma advises, "Go and sit under a tree..." The tree signifies a saint, a truly enlightened person who can lead one to God. "Saints may be compared to a tree: they always point upwards and grant shade and shelter to all. They are free from likes and dislikes and whoever seeks refuge in them, wholeheartedly, will find peace." She adds, "Just as water cleanses everything by its mere contact, even so the sight, touch, blessing, nay the very Remembrance of a real sadhu, little by little, clears away all impure desires and longings."

Often people discount the idea or belief, that an external Guru is necessary. They tout, "My Guru is inside me." To which I respond, "Yes it is." Everything is inside of you. Every frequency of light, every note of the Song of the Divine. But if I ask you to sing an F above middle C, can you do it? Do you have enough clarity, enough awareness to be able to pick a specific frequency out of the ether amongst all the other noises in the internal, and external world? I can't. Yet. But if you sing me an F, I can mirror it back to you with no problem, then I can practice connecting to that note even after you have gone, until the world of noise once again takes over and I need you to sing it to me again. This is the role of an outer Guru. They can sing, embody, emanate, vibrate at the note of human potential so that you can calibrate, and mirror, and aspire to sing that note even when you are alone. And one day you will be, and when you can then sing that note, emanate that frequency all on your own, isolate, tap into and consciously live from that frequency, then your Guru Tattwa will have been burning brightly inside of you too.

In the same truth that everything is inside you, the knowledge of how to perform open-heart surgery is also inside of you. And yet, you would not boast to be able to do this without the proper training, without the proper teachers and mentors for this endeavor. Spiritual life is no different. We need to humble ourselves to admit that even while everything is inside of us, knowing it, embodying it and consciously living it are vastly different things. We all need training, guidance, mentoring and tutoring in whatever skill we are endeavoring to "Re-member".

So there is a leap of faith and a humbling that happens when the personality/ego starts to loosen its vocabulary on what is "true" and what is "reality", and starts to let the soul's mysterious unfathomable "other worldly" experiences take equal stage with the intellect. Some call this imagination, but for me, there is a difference between imagining something that is not there - which I do all the time, and being willing to get so quiet and so subtle, that you start to experience things that others may not be able to relate to. It is part of waking up, expanding your awareness, and Re-membering your essential Self while engaging with this three dimensional reality.

If your heart has experienced this other worldly, multi dimensional, magical, unexplainable event in the presence of an Enlightened one, a Master (and when I say Master I mean they have mastered themselves, not the master *over* anyone else) then you understand what I am talking about. If you have not, then it probably sounds a little far-fetched and unrelatable. For when it comes down to it, it is like trying to explain an orgasm to a virgin. There are no words that can truly describe it. Just prepare yourself for a mutually respectful, kind and loving relationship and be open to it when it happens.

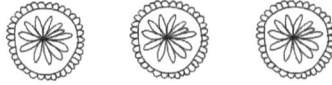

✿   ✿   ✿

A few days before the end of my first trip to the Ashram we were called to 'Darshan'. Darshan, is the opportunity to have sight of something, or someone who embodies the Light. An electric murmur went through our group, as it suddenly felt like Christmas eve, and we had just got the television update that Santa was indeed on his way. Apparently "Sri Swamiji" or great Swami, had not given Darshan for quite some time and we were very blessed to be granted an audience. Now, you may be detecting a slight tone of irreverence in my words; and you would be right. I had never met anyone truly worthy, in my humble opinion, of reverence. Respect, sure, more as a cultural obligation, but I had never met anyone who was empowered within themselves, and who did not request to have power over me, or anyone else. I didn't trust anyone, and would not be bowing down, just because everyone else did.

After waiting in line, oscillating between feeling like we were going to see the headmaster and our fairy Godfather, we were ushered into the room where He was sitting. There sat an old man, perched on a cushion on a wooden bed frame. He was thin, bordering frail in the shoulders, but with a little belly protruding from his unadorned terracotta coloured korta[8] and pale. He didn't look like he got out much, nor cared to. The frailness of his body, and the simplicity of his appearance seemed to amplify the contrast of the air of command he had about him. It was a strength you could not mess with, but it did not protrude outwards. It was like sitting in front of a 300 year old Redwood tree. One that really

---

[8] Korta: A loose fitting, thigh length top, short or long sleeves with no buttons.

didn't care if you took shelter in its branches. Its leaves were focused on the sun, its foundation communing with the depths of the Earth. You could throw anything you wanted at it and it wouldn't budge. It wouldn't even notice, like the Fool card of the Tarot who is so intoxicated with Love that he walks straight off the cliff. We, on the other hand had put on the nicest cleanest clothes we had, dressing to the ashram nines, our energy, ok, my energy, being more of a gnat.

There was an air of decorum about him, people sitting closest to him knew their place around him, but as the rings of acquaintance blossomed out there was an undertone of uneasiness. 'What do I say? Is he really enlightened? How will I know he's not a fake? Will he perform a siddhi or power to prove to us he's enlightened? Is this what I came to the other side of the world for, an old man on a wooden bench?'

He started by talking about the temperature a room should be when you practice asana. How he had asked for our fans in our rooms to be disconnected as to make us slightly uncomfortable - "it's easier to transform when you are slightly uncomfortable" he said and assured us he could afford the electricity bill.

He spoke seeming nonchalant pleasantries for 10 - 15 minutes, and then, in my memory at least, he seemed to stop mid sentence and close his eyes. A ripple of uneasiness went through the room. 'What's he doing? Is he asleep? The saint is Narcoleptic! What are we supposed to do? Everyone is sitting with their eyes closed, ok I'll do that, pretend I'm meditating, try not to move, oh my god my foot is asleep, try not to MOVE! You're a Yoga teacher for Christ sake, you should be able to sit for 30 minutes without moving! You're a fake, if you move they will all know you're a FAKE!'

And then, like a mirror briefly catching the sunlight, something shiny flashed across my consciousness. I felt something, as small as a mosquito, and as fluttery as a butterfly. Not intrusive, but curious, it came though the top of my head, hovered, then continued down my spine, stopping at different points down my back then continuing to move down and back up.

One part panic, but two parts fascination brushed over me. My mind started to wonder, 'Don't move, could it be? Is that You? Are You doing this? Are you checking me out? This should be creepy, but it's not. What? You see? What do you see? Oh my god, you see me? NO! Don't look! What? Really? It's ok? But do you know I've done this? You do? Do you know I've done that? A-ha? Do you realize this is what my mind thinks about? What I'm capable of? Really? And you see everything I can be? Will be? Have the potential to be? And what? What's that? It's ok? You understand? You have nothing but Love for me?' Memory flooded my senses, images, feelings, different times of my life. 'Hold on, I remember this feeling, in dark ally ways as I walked home in the city, in the depths of my panic attacks, at the root of my despair, it was You, it was You who was always there.' And then as disconcertingly as it arrived, it flew out the top of my head and a feeling of pure Love washed over me, rendering me incapable of another thought.

My mind was completely blank. Sri Swamiji, this old man sitting in front of me, opened his eyes and looked around the room and concluded the meeting. The room abuzz, there were sideways glances portraying that he had simultaneously looked at everyone, but no one wanted to say it out loud, the feeling that everyone had been touched by pure unconditional Love. Did everyone have a *"butterskitto"* experience? He did not look at me, but without a doubt in my mind he saw me, the fullness of my potential and flaws, more completely than I have ever seen myself. And all I felt was a quiet unwavering Love.

I walked out of that room that day understanding why people renounce, why they bow down, why they humble themselves in his presence. I understood that the perspective and the frequency of light that he fully embodied was the potential of the human race and perhaps even beyond. That he was a living example of what it was to realize oneSelf, to be God intoxicated. To have the ability to look at all as One, to see one as All, known in sanskrit as Atmabhav, and to offer nothing but Love, Compassion, and Blessings. Everyone that day was offered blessings, but it was up to us to utilize them to their fullest. For me, there was nothing left to do but commit to getting as close to that potential in this life time as I can. Now, I may never get anywhere close to what he was able to embody, but I have seen what is possible, and so long as in my heart, and His eyes, I am going in the right direction, I will have succeeded.

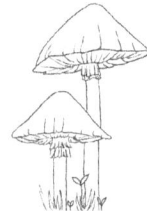

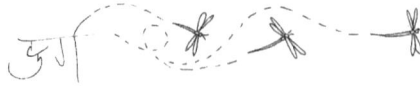

FIVE

- A Prayer and a Promise- part one

At some point you have to ask yourself, is this note, this frequency of thought that I am engaged with right now what I want to be dominating my life song? If it is, great! If it is not, then you have to find something to attune your inner song to. You need to dream a frequency that you can calibrate your being with. We all do it, knowingly or not, in the company we keep, the music we listen to, the food we eat, every action we partake in, is a calibration. Sometimes we calibrate to the shadows and suffering of life, drugs, addiction, alcohol, in the hopes it will miraculously quell the pain inside, or we can calibrate to the light, and allow our own shadows to be brought to the surface and at each moment choose, choose the note, that we will tether our life force to.

We all have aspects of our life that we find challenging, some more debilitating than others. Some patterns, karmas, experiences, we just can't quite figure out how to disconnect from and in turn establish a new pattern to embody. As Rita Mae Brown, the mystery novelist, wrote in her 1983 book "Sudden Death",

"Insanity is doing the same thing over and over again and expecting different results."[9]

To acknowledge that we are not, and don't necessarily know how to, changing some of our more challenging patterns that repeatedly induce bouts of suffering in our lives is a liberating step to shifting that which seems too hard to digest. To admit that, until

---

[9] "Insanity" quote often mis attributed to Albert Einstein

this point, all we have known is how to maneuver through this life from the perspective of controlling, doing, needing, taking and accumulating, then maybe surrender, being, aspiring, serving and giving is what we need to do. Maybe cultivating these qualities will help us to yield different results from our actions. But to jump-start this transition we need Grace, we need blessings, we need help. When our egoic cup is full, to bring in a new frequency, we must offer something. This is the Divine law. The more we offer, the more we can receive. If we want to pray, we need to promise. In order to receive from the Divine, we need to offer something. So we need to be careful what we wish for, we need to make sure what our heart beats for, is truly worthy of our sacrifice.

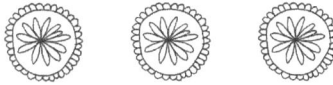

In the early fall of 2007, when my teaching career in Vancouver was in full swing I was invited to a few opportunities to partake in external substances to help stimulate an internal experience. I was never a huge fan of recreational drugs, but had on occasion tried something here and there. Gratefully, nothing ever stuck into a habit or a lifestyle, nor did it ever come close to the kind of connected experience I had had in Sri Swamiji's presence. So on this particular Saturday night, we were gathering to worship Ma Ayahuasca in downtown Vancouver. I had only participated in one other Ayahuasca ceremony before where I experienced great sweetness and devastating lows, sometimes simultaneously. This night however, there was no great purging, or soul splitting emotional releases, just the guy in the sleeping bag next to me whose constant rustling sounded like a torrent of cockroaches were about to scuttle over me at any moment. Yet, somewhere amongst the anticipation of complete bug creep out, a simple message came forth that reverberated through me as though my insides were made of stone, "You have an out in Tibet if you want it."

These words, echoed in my being through the feathered dream of the Mother's womb and into the rigid and austere light of day. "You have an out in Tibet." I had just spent the last three months planning and paying for my trip that was to take me from China, through Tibet and into Nepal and then down to the Ashram for a month of Seva. The trip was coming up fast and I intuitively knew I was being shown that within life we have natural portals, legitimate off ramps that we can utilize if our soul is feeling that it does not want to continue this trajectory, in this lifetime. This is not suicide. It's not a conscious deciding to get off the merry go round in the delusion that all my patterns would be neutralized, but a breath in my soul's story with the knowledge that I would have to keep digesting this karmic pie at another time. My soul was being given, one could say, prior knowledge of an astrologically appropriate comma. Either way, life after Tibet was never going to be the same, with or without my body attached.

I turned to the only person I knew that could hold this information in the same light that I was perceiving it, my teacher Anandashakti-ji. I called her in Toronto to download my experience, hoping I could bounce off her a barometer of, am I being crazy, or I should take this seriously? She did not answer. The message I left her voicemail was very conscious of not mentioning Ayahuasca, or the message I had received while in ceremony. I simply asked her to call me back at her earliest convenience, with a tinge of desperation in my voice.

Upon hearing my voice on her voicemail, her eyes locked on the time on the dash of her car. It was 1:08pm her time, 108 being an auspicious number to a yogi, and as she listened to my voice she too intuitively was given the same very clear message, "Shivani has an out in Tibet."

When she returned my call I relayed the whole experience and we decided the best cause of action would be for her to get on a plane and come to Vancouver to help me decide what to do.

What a gift! To have the opportunity to really consciously decide to live, something we have every day and yet do not recognize nor utilize it. We merely survive until tomorrow. And to have someone whom I trusted and loved come to help me really decide. For this was no flippant decision. There had been so many times in my 27 years to that point that I didn't want to be alive anymore. Much of my life up to then I had experienced tremendous anxiety, depression, self abuse, emotional abuse and emotional pain through very challenging circumstances.

Yet, I didn't take this message as being an opportunity to leave behind all that had been painful, more, I felt it was an opportunity to get real, to focus on the light, rather than try and survive the darkness. To dream, fully and completely, of what I might be capable of, what might be capable of coming through me, if I had the right support, guidance and was able to cleanly and completely surrender to this potential.

It was an opportunity to consciously open to Grace.

Meeting Sri Swamiji the year before had lit something in me, a light that everything in my reality started to be filtered through. I realized that the human life could be so much more than what I was experiencing, and yet, on the third Dimensional level my rational mind kept reminding me that my experience was, well, pretty much all in my head and heart. Reality was, I had sat in the presence of something, someone that was *in*, but not *of*, this world, for one hour. That's it. To the mind, my mind at least, this is not a lot to base your whole life trajectory on. Yet, to my heart what Sri Swamiji embodied was the realest and only tangible thing my heart wanted to ever engage with or move towards.

It was clear that if I was going to stay in body, on this earth plane, then I needed help. Real tangible help. To surrender, to let go of all the pain from before, and to step forward. There was only one person that I felt could take on a piece of work like me - Sri Swamiji. I knew harnessing this message and consciously dreaming a new life would require me to completely surrender my control of where my life was leading, and yet, a single seed of desire would not let go; I wanted a family.

I wanted to share my life with a husband my equal or better in every way. To know what it was to be in right relationship with the masculine, something that had eluded my life thus far. What it was to be physically and wholeheartedly loved by a man, that was in himself walking the same path. And I wanted a child. Everything else, my mind could walk away from if it needed to. But these two would not budge. So, after days of soul searching, conversations, layers of fear, excitement, anticipation, and tears, I lit a candle on my alter and uttered words from the deepest part of my being.

"Divine Mother, Beloved Sri Swamiji, I acknowledge that I have an out from this lifetime on my upcoming trip to Tibet and in looking at my life so far I cannot continue to live in this way, with these patterns. Yet I feel, that given the opportunity, and with your guidance there is something beautiful that can come through me in time. I need help. So if I stay in body, I surrender. To you. From this moment on, I promise, my life is in your hands, everything I will do, will be to be closer to you. To embody the light that you have shown me is possible. It is no longer my life, it is your will through me. I don't want to go another moment in this life without you. And I humbly pray that you bless me with a husband and child to share this experience with. My heart seems to be able to let go of everything else, but this. By your Grace. In humility, Hari Om Tat Sat"

Tibet was not what I expected. I went there with the intention of Re-membering a lost piece of my soul. But all I felt was sparks of light engulfed in great shadow. I snuck into monasteries where the monks were in training for debate. I sat in their courtyards while they chanted. Willing myself to be a tree, or blend with the wall, hoping the white woman wouldn't stand out and cause a disturbance and an invitation to leave. Inside these places there was a vibrant-ness to their clothes, to the tress, while outside of those very walls oppression and hardship made it hard to breathe.

There are two words that plague the mind of any traveller through Tibet: altitude sickness. Surprisingly, I was not as affected as my travelling partners were. I stayed in good health and was able to explore, while they were confined to a bed or short walks outside. One night we became stranded in a town in the middle of nowhere after being turned back by the Chinese at Everest base camp where we were intending to sleep. Aside from one of our travelling mates whispering menacingly to my friend that he could kill us right here tonight and no one would ever know what happened, there was no real drama, for me, on the whole trip that would have foretold a death.

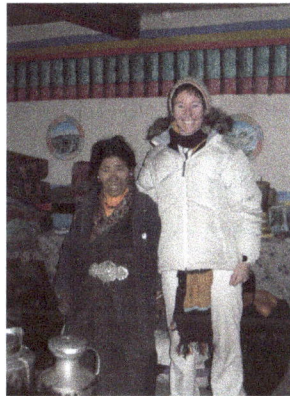

The Gracious lady that gave us shelter after being turned back by the Chinese authorities.

Well, except maybe the road out of Tibet. That was definitely a death-defying experience in the literal sense. It was a thin snake squeezed between a shear cliff of terror, and avalanche tunnels held up with two-by-fours reinforced with prayers. I believe I actually super humanly held my breath for three hours straight, all the way to the boarder of Nepal. Kathmandu was a discombobulating bouncing between prayer flags and wifi. Neither looking like they were supposed to be there, and subsequently neither was I. So, I bussed through the countryside with 100 other people in a 40 seater bus, to Kalompong in northern India where its people captured a piece of my heart through their bonds of community and simplicity in life. But I was eager to keep moving like a river, who after a long journey can finally hear the waves of the ocean, to the abode of my beloved Sri Swamiji, and a month of seva in the Ashram.

For me, Ashram life is a dance of light always weaving its experience for your growth. Both *pleasant and unpleasant* experiences feel, in the very least, supported and guided. It makes it easier to step back and watch the leela, or play, play out.

Unfortunately, upon arriving in the Ashram for the Yajnas[10] that year, I became very ill with bronchitis. Fever, cough, hard to breathe; the type of experience that up in Tibet, when combined with the high elevations could easily have turned into pneumonia and much more serious consequences, even death. I did my best to continue my Karma yoga, serving food to the Yajna participants, cutting vegetables in the kitchen and cleaning the Puja area.

Even in my bronchial stupor, I jumped in head first into the swift river that is Ashram life. Giving my all to the tasks I was assigned and trying to take in all of the programs and rituals that were happening around me. Consciously, the bronchitis was playing out to be my physical purification as part of my choice, my soul's choice to stay in body and clear out old patterns that had haunted my being for years. Simultaneously, on a soul level, there was a light that was being called in, that the Holy was being fed, and that it was recalibrating me and planting seeds in my soul that I can't even begin to comprehend.

---

[10] Yajna: Yajna literally means "sacrifice, devotion, worship, offering", and refers in Hinduism to any ritual done in front of a sacred fire, often with mantras. Yajna has been a Vedic tradition, described in a layer of Vedic literature called Brahmanas, as well as Yajurveda. The tradition has evolved from offering oblations and libations into sacred fire to symbolic offerings in the presence of sacred fire. - Wikipedia

During this Yajna, the proceedings were presided by both Sw Niranjanananda and Sw Satyasangananda, who we affectionately call Sw. Niranjan and Sw Satsangi. Sri Swamiji only coming into the area of the festivities and Puja on the last day, having wanted to focus people's main attention on the guest of honour, Devi. I have always perceived Sw Niranjan and Sw Satsangi as being the right and left hand, the action organs, of Sri Swamiji's heart. Sri Swamiji himself referring to them as his Manas Putra[11] and Sankalpa Putra[12] respectively. While these three beings are encased in different bodies, and are filtered through different personalities, at their essence, I perceive them as embodiments and expressions of the same frequency.

While most of our experiences in life fall away with no value, like what you had for lunch last Tuesday, seemingly innate experiences in the presence of Masters seem to get etched into your soul as though they are predetermined déjà vu's that are required to be remembered and to be recalled into the mind medicinally in times of sorrow or suffering. These, often brief, and outwardly inconsequential interactions seem to hold layers and layers of digestion as one evolves.

It's fascinating to me, to consider the different levels of *dimensional perception* of different people all interacting simultaneously in the same space, and yet with all the karmas and samskaras bouncing off each other it is clear that what we are experiencing on the surface as reality, is not the same as what these Swami's are experiencing, and the conscious awareness of this, to them, is amusing. I can't help but wonder what it is like to be in their "chappals[13]". Not easy, I imagine, everybody around them constantly, and sometimes unconsciously vying for their attention,

---

[11] Manas Putra: Child born of ones mind or thought.

[12] Sankalpa Putra: Child born of ones intention.

[13] Chappals: Shoes

for blessings, for a reprieve from their suffering. But I can only project my own limited awareness onto what I see and perceive, which of course, is like being plankton on a whale's back wondering what it's like to be the Ocean.

Mornings start early during a Yajna. Sometimes the kitchen is chopping vegetables at 3 or 4 am. It's a lot of peas to peel by hand when your making lunch for three thousand people! I would often try and get a few minutes in morning program before I was due at my turn to serve breakfast at 8am. Eking out every last minute in front of the Devi before I needed to step into Seva. On one such morning as I got up to leave, there was only a very small pathway leading through the crowd to the small archway out of the compound that ran next to a concrete ledge a foot off the ground. The whole area was teaming with people, and navigating the swells of movement was challenging at best. As I decided to dash through a small opening along the path Sw. Niranjan, at that exact moment started walking towards me. I stopped like a deer in headlights. Do I squeeze past? Do I back up the long path delaying my arrival at my duty by several minutes? or... I decided to hop up on the ledge and walk towards him where we would be able to pass each other without touching. But as soon as got up on it, I realized that by standing I would be taller than him, which didn't feel right, so I crouched down like a duck walking a tight rope balancing on the ledge past him. Quacking a quick "Namo Narayana" to him as we passed each other. While awash with embarrassment, I was not late to seva!

My experience of Sw. Niranjanananda is that he is a being of intense light. A light that can take a room as dark as night and flood it into daylight just by walking into the space. A light that can also be focused so acutely that it can burn through your ignorance like a laparoscopic laser. This light is encased as a tall, elegant man who has been wholeheartedly dedicated to the Tradition of Sannyas and the Sankalpa of his Guru, Sri Swamiji since his conception. He is completely present, and so totally in the moment, in every moment, that he can dance between being utterly childlike and playful, with a smile that encapsulates all the joy in the world into one gesture, and in the blink of an eye can cast a look that feels like Shiva himself seeking and destroying ignorance like the oracle in the Never-ending Story, and never be out of sync with the right action of the Divine's dance.

During one of my lunch serving duties I was collecting my buckets of food that were about to be served to the hungry people waiting behind their banana leaf plates as they sat on the ground on long rolled mats, and I realized I had everything bar the rice. Feeling the pressure of having everything go smoothly, as I could see that others sections were starting to eat, while my line of 100 people or so were pleading at me with hunger in their eyes. I spun around in utter frustration and exclaimed angrily, to no one in particular, "WHERE'S THE RICE?!" Instead of my eyes landing on the empty buckets, they landed on two feet. Slowly my eyes travelled up a very tall figure and rested on Sw Niranjan's face who was standing not two feet away, silently watching me throwing a tantrum. Blush is not really an accurate colour describing this moment, more hot coal glow just before it disintegrates into ash. I turned and ran to the kitchen to find the rice and bring it back so that the line of people I was serving could eat. Rice however was about a 5-10 minute wait, and when I came back with it there was Sw Niranjan standing half way down the line, talking and laughing, entertaining, and distracting the line of hungry people while they waited for their lunch, for many in this line this was their *soul* meal of the day. Complete gratitude washed over me, having expected to come back to find people disgruntled and 'hangry', they were not in the least interested in lunch. Only Him. And while he never looked or acknowledged me in anyway, I always felt that he had been there to help a sincere glitch in the proceedings to bide time while we waited for the rice to be ready.

As loud and bolshie as I am at times, I have come to appreciate Grace's subtle and delicate qualities. It is quiet. It does not have a pointing sign that says "look here!" It gives, and it waits, and it sings an almost inaudible tune. But when you can hear that song, see its gift, its guidance, - often only in hindsight - Grace is activated into reality. Grace looks mundane on the surface, but if there is one thing I have learnt in this journey, there is magic every day, every moment, and the only reason we can't see it is because WE are not looking. We are not always living a life attuned to its song. We are distracted. We are singing loudly and out of tune all the while complaining that we can't hear the rose bud open.

Cleaning the Puja area in the Ashram is a blessing for anyone with the opportunity, but for anyone who knows me, cleaning is not always something I naturally do with full heart, to put it mildly. While my western stiff hips didn't always enjoy taking a wet rag and scrubbing what seemed like endless marble, what looks like on the surface like cleaning a floor, is really an extra blessing of an internal cleaning of yourSelf. While cleaning we hold silence, which allows you to really feel the different aspects of the Puja area. From the Panch Agni area where Sri Swamiji did his Sadhana, Murtis (statues) of Krishna or Durga to the Rudra Tree where Shiva sits surrounded by the lingams of consciousness. It was here, one morning, at the foot of Shiva, while on my hands and knees washing the floor that I got a glimpse of feet standing about three feet from me. Trying to do the look, don't look, awkward dance of someone star-struck, I realized Sri Swaimiji, Sw Niranjan and Sw Satsangi were all standing right there in front of me. There were engaged in a discussion in Hindi, so naturally, I didn't understand a single thing, but it seemed that Sri Swamiji was giving some instruction to Sw Niranjan and Sw Satsangi for the future by the way he was standing with his hands on his hips, leaning slightly back and pointing to something little ways from us. While it felt like an hour, they must have been there for only a minute or two. And while on this earth plane they never looked at me, that I could see, or had any physical interaction. I was merely the person on the cleaning team washing the marble floor. They came, stood, chatted in Hindi, and walked away. Or so I thought...

So there I was, had survived the Yajnas with bronchitis, served and gave all that I could and held my prayer and a promise in my heart each day that I was there, but so what?

Internally I had said a prayer and made a promise to the Divine, to a man, a Guru, whom I have only been in the presence of twice. A man who has never spoken to me directly. I have made an internal, nevertheless, heart pounding declaration of surrender. And yet, I wonder, does the absence of it being spoken out loud, or having never been acknowledged outwardly by anyone or any of the three guides of our lineage in this 'reality' make it less valid? And then, on the night before I left, homeward bound, I had a dream.

First of all though, let me give you a bit of background. Have you ever been talking to someone in a kind and honest communication and then the hair on the both parties' arms stand up on end? And you feel that whatever that was just said between the two of you was something to take notice of? It denotes a shift of frequency in the connection between you from a mundane chitchat to, "Hey! This is important! Take notice!" This shift of frequency in waking state is a wonderful barometer as to if I am on the right track.

Similarly, dreams also have different frequencies. Some dreams are a discharge of excess energy or memories that need to be processed and discarded, similar to defragmenting your hard drive on your computer. Other dreams have a prophetic quality to them.

Lucid dreaming has the experience of knowing you are asleep, and experiencing something consciously as a soul, without a physical body, in any dimensional reality. And then I have had dreams where I'm interacting with an enlightened Master. These dreams, again, have a different frequency to them, the frequency that while it's still in a mundane dream setting, the master you are dreaming with is consciously interacting with you in your dream. What is said and done in this space is conscious to them in the waking state. It is for this reason that on the rare and beautiful occasions that I have had the opportunity to experience a dream with any Master I have always taken note and taken very seriously the message and tone of the interactions conveyed. For in working with dreams, how you feel in the interaction in the dream has as much weight as what is said. Something we can also aspire to in our more waking states! In my experience, there are certain Masters that prefer to interact with Sadhaks[14] from a dream place for it does not have the messy outward ego stories attached to it, and it has the tone of a private inner relationship with the Guru Tattwa or Frequency of light that holds truth.

So towards the end of my 2007 stay in the Ashram, while I was still in the throws of my earthly purification through bronchitis, I had a dream that I have always remembered, and many times taken solace in for trusting my path in a world that is so fickle in its relationship to Faith. To me, it was an acknowledgement of my prayer and promise being accepted and the encouragement to go home and keep walking forward.

There I was standing in a concert arena. The kind that only the biggest music stars play, U2, Madonna and the like. I've done this many times in my days of working with the music industry, so it was not an unfamiliar setting to me, in any state. My love of music had given me purpose for many years, my love of the music industry?

---

14 Seeker on the path of enlightenment

Not so much. This arena was empty of people, just the gear for an upcoming concert was there, I had no idea for who.

Arenas are like wombs, more, incubators of plastic, metal and concrete. Where something living will come and birth into something beautiful, but it, in and of itself is sterile and uninviting. Beside me stood Sri Swamiji. We stood there for a moment looking at the vast space and then he put his hand on my back over my spleen, guiding me to walk forward into the middle of the space. We weaved our way through rows and sections until we arrived at the most optimal spot in the whole place for sound quality. The engineer's soundboard. As he sat me down at the desk, I started to protest that I had no right being there, that any second someone was going to come and yell at me for being in a place I had no right being, that maybe I could move over slightly onto a seat of the audience. "No!" he said standing beside me, "you will go where I put you, and no one will bother you if you are doing what I have asked you to do. You stay here."

And suddenly I was back in the Ashram. The feeling over me was calm, strong, protected and encouraged. Some digging into the symbology and frequency of the spleen, bought forth the relationship of action of "Thy will", where as the liver is more the frequency of "my will". So, I will be put where He wants me to be; let thy will be done.

Bronchitis stayed with me for my whole stay in the Ashram that year. I was so sick that someone in the Ashram offered to pay for me to stay in a very nice hotel in Kolkata for a night to help me rest before my long flights home. This, I now feel, was also was at the energetic prompting of Sri Swamiji, always taking care of our needs, not placating to our wants. I boarded the plane in a fevered daze, I slept, coughed and wheezed for most of the plane ride home, utterly miserable as only one can be when sick and travelling large distances alone. And yet, upon setting foot in Canada, not once did I cough again, fever was gone, the future was upon me.

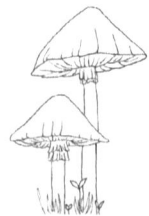

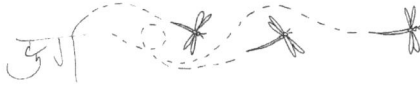

SIX

- The Bird and the Bees

"Your pain is the breaking of the shell
that encloses your understanding.
Even as the stone of the fruit must break, that its heart may stand in
the sun, so must you know pain. And could you keep your heart in
wonder at the daily miracles of your life, your pain would not seem
less wondrous than your joy;
And you would accept the seasons of your heart, even as you have
always accepted the seasons that pass over your fields.
And you would watch with serenity
through the winters of your grief."

The Prophet, Kahlil Gibran

I've always appreciated the cartoon where there is a group of people standing listening to a person speak from a podium at the front of the room. The speaker asks, "Who wants change?!" And everyone puts up their hand, and in the next frame the speakers asks, "Who wants to change?!" And not a single hand is raised.

Pain is life's trumped song announcing irrevocable change.

It's a birthing song. The book ending to grief's Westing[15] song of Gratitude. It's the royal trumpets heralding a new chapter in this soul's journey. It's how all good stories begin. Suffering, on the other hand, is the inability to honour pain for what she is. It is

---

[15] Westing: is an ancient Egyptian term for leaving, or dying.

the whaling of change being rejected in the way a sapling tries to hold back a broken dam. I say she, for it is the Divine feminine, Shakti, which stimulates change, transformation, evolution. She pushes the portals open both in the things we humans call births and deaths. These seemingly definite boundaries which are but commas in the soul's journey through a lucid dream. Often humbling, pain demands the ego to step off centre stage for a deeper part of us to come to the surface and be integrated, a peeling away of what we no longer need, to grow, and a Re-membering of what/who/we are.

Often in life's hindsight, it is the painful periods that in fact show us our own birthing while still in body. Multiple births, initiations, opportunities for leaps in consciousness, the discarding of the old ways of being, and emerging into the new, can happen while embodying the same meat suit. After all, from the point of view of the babe, birthing from the mother's womb and "into the world" is but a shift of consciousness. The world was always there, but the babe was not able to perceive it yet, or at best had a distorted perception of it. It is this process that happens again and again as we walk a path of spirituality. For our ignorant and asleep state, besotted with Maya, the dream we call life, is but a distorted perception of the Divine which is not 'out there' but 'right here' and we are here to live through these initiations, not just learn about them.

So it is not surprising that one of the first teachings I learnt from Anandashakti when stepping onto the path of Yoga was, "Believe nothing except your own direct experience." Study, learn, don't disregard the teachings because you don't relate, but have discernment. Don't just believe blindly about something because someone tells you this is the right way, always bounce it off your own heart to see where you sit with it. It's important to learn the teachings, but the objective is to experience them. To see how these nuggets of wisdom actually start to manifest in your life as you gain awareness, and peel back the layers of conditioning that are not your optimal Self.

A direct experience is of course, every moment of every day. From the mundane to miracles. They are all moments that give you the opportunity to heal or shine. They are all moments to help you Re-member who you are, beyond ego, beyond "you". Remember...

Sometimes the most traumatic experiences of our lives are also our biggest gifts. To make this change from a story of trauma to gift comes through the willingness to change your perception. After all, Yoga is not about changing your reality, it's about changing the perspective and perception of your reality. It's about expanding your consciousness from the doer, to the witness and beyond. To dissolve the attachments of good and bad. This comes from much awareness, sometimes a lot of hard work, but always with the magic of Grace and Divine Blessings.

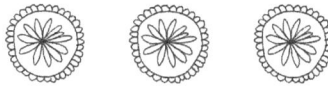

❀ ❀ ❀

When I was twenty-one I was diagnosed with severe Endometriosis, *"Endo" is an often painful disorder in which tissue that normally lines the inside of your uterus — the endometrium — grows outside your uterus. Endometriosis most commonly involves your ovaries, fallopian tubes and the tissue lining your pelvis.*[16] It's considered, at least when I was diagnosed, "incurable" and can create so much scar tissue that it makes it hard to conceive a child.

The degree to which I experienced this disease meant that I was given three choices. Have a hysterectomy, go through six months of drug-induced menopause and/or have laparoscopic surgeries every year and a half to two years to keep it "under

---

[16] https://en.wikipedia.org/wiki/Endometriosis

control." The medical system in the early 2000's didn't know what causes it, and didn't know how to fix it beyond a band aid.

Which is why six months into my nine month yoga teacher training, after menopause and three surgeries in four years did nothing, when my surgeon couldn't find a single trace of the disease, I started to become a "believer" in this whole Yoga thing. Even though I no longer had any symptoms of the disease currently, the extent of scar tissue from the years previous meant that I had a very slim chance of ever getting pregnant.

Six months after I returned to Vancouver from my life-altering trip to India, via Tibet, I met my beloved, the man I was going to marry, and naturally, children came into conversation pretty quickly. We decided that we would actively try for a year and see what happened. Failing that, we would adopt. I was nervous and skeptical, having been told for years that conceiving might be a long and harrowing ordeal, repeatedly being told by the medical professionals not to hold my breath. As pregnancy and childbirth were a topic I had only heard about in terms of pain, dying, fear and at the end, if you're lucky, a healthy babe, I decided to start reprogramming my mind into being open to possibilities, while simultaneously surrendering to the most high.

It was in December of that year that I, along with some students, went back to Sri Swamiji's Ashram, Rikhia, for a month of Karma Yoga and to experience Yog Poornima Yajna; the Yajna that is performed after Sita Kalyanams Yajna to Devi which is dedicated to Shiva, the Masculine principle. I returned to the Ashram with the book "Ina May's Guide to Childbirth", a whisper of hope that if one half of my prayer had already manifested then surely the other could too, and some hair to wrap around the fertility tree in Kolkata's Kali temple for good measure.

The first day of our trip I was asked to choose five of the students I had brought with me to come and attend to Sri Swamiji's rock garden outside his private residence. Excitedly we followed the Swami in and started work. It was serene, silent, surreal. I was pretty sure Sri Swamiji was in his house, even though I never saw him.

As I wiped each leaf clear of the lime that had splattered while the wall behind had been recently painted, a bird flying out of a big tree not 10 meters from me caught my eye. I watched it spread its wings and fly away and then I didn't give it a second thought. A few minutes later Sarah (not her real name), was asked to go and get a brick from the other side of the garden. She did, and as she walked back, she started to swat at her hair. She thought there was a single bee buzzing around her, but we could see that the bird had disturbed a whole hive and there were hundreds of bees starting to swarm and sting her.

Knowing that the woman standing next to me, Mandy (also, not her real name), was deathly allergic by a single bee sting and seeing Sarah start to panic, I dropped my tools and ran over to her. I grabbed her by her arms and told her to hold her breath. I dunked her in a barrel of water trying to drown the bees so they would stop stinging her. As she came up for air I told her to run and turned to dunk myself in the barrel for by this time, I too was being attacked. To my disgust there was a film of bees an inch thick lying on top of the water; there was no way I was going in there, so I started to panic. As I turned to run, Mandy told me later that all she could see was my whole neck black with bees.

If you have ever been attacked by a swarm of bees you will know that you can't see them... only hear them. So I also started to run. Swearing like a sailor, to Sri Swamiji, *at* Sri Swamiji, at anyone. Thoughts running through my mind — "If he was so omnipresent, compassionate, enlightened, how could he let this happen? On his own front doorstep!"

I thought maybe if I yelled my mantra out loud that they would magically disappear. This was not the case...

I ran across the whole compound to a small swimming pool hoping to jump in, but it was empty. So I turned again and made it to the Puja area before multiple Swami's started to run towards me with a blanket. They would throw it on me, trapping bees with me under the blanket, I would throw it off. Then they would throw it on me again. I got ushered into a bathroom by a female Swami, she hastily stripped my clothes off... and bees that were trapped in them went flying everywhere. Re-clothed and with no bees left on my body I was taken to the meeting room where Sarah was sitting. Both of us in tears, both of us completely in shock.

Two Swamis, each with tweezers, sat and picked out the stingers. They counted around eighty bee stings on each of us. Welts covering our necks, hands, eye lids, up our noses, on our scalp, in our mouths, ears, arms, and feet.

They had two doctors on the grounds to come and check us and gave us the option of going to see someone outside the Ashram for a second opinion. My only question was if I was going to have a life threatening reaction. They said that if I hadn't by then, it was unlikely, so I opted to stay put.

As the Swamis finished picking out the stings, someone trying to console me, suggested I perform the healing breath called Bhramari, the humming bee breath. She was met with a filthy look of bewilderment. I could see the genuine concern and rattling that this had bought into the Ashram - it's not every day that a woman dressed head to toe in yellow, yelling and screaming obscenities like a sailor would run through the sacred and silent Puja area.

All I could think of while I sat there swinging between shock and hysteria was that nothing ever bad would happen outside His front door step. I couldn't and wouldn't believe that this was a terrible thing happening. It was going to be the best thing that ever happened to me, I just didn't understand it yet. And simply put, it was.

Wrapped in blankets, the four other students walked in along with the Swami that was gardening with us. Mandy, with wide eyes and herself in shock, told me, "I didn't know what to do, so I knelt down next to the wall. Put my hand on it to keep myself as still as I could, and started to say my mantra silently. All these bees were flying around my head, then flying into the wall and dying. Not one touched me, I could feel this force field coming off me and not one touched me."

With the stings removed and the venom starting to affect our bodies we were taken back to our room. For six hours we rotated from the squat toilet with diarrhea, to a bucket for vomiting. Then we passed out with fevers.

The next morning I dreaded even leaving our room. Everyone would know, everyone was looking, everyone was talking. I looked like I had overdone it on Botox. No wrinkles on my forehead, no eyelids, huge lips and hands. Everything was swollen and I still had a fever.

A wave of whispers ran between people's lips like they were trying to pass rose petals from one to another. We were being invited to Darshan with Sri Swamiji. Too weak to stand in the line to wait to go into Ganesh Kutir, I sat on the concrete, knees tucked under my chin. After being ushered in with about 50 other people Sri Swamiji asked me to introduce the group I had brought with me. I couldn't remember their names and had to be prompted for each one. Then, when they opened up the floor for questions, something "now or never" burst forth from me.

I wanted to ask about The Great White Brotherhood, a collective of souls whom he had offered thanks to in the forward of one of his books, Meditations on the Tantras. Why I wanted to know about this now when I could hardly stand up I'll never understand, but in that moment, I couldn't remembered which book it was in and as I tried in vain to describe which book it was, people around me started to get frustrated. Comments that I was wasting Sri Swamiji's time were called across the room, suggestions that he should move on to another question were offered. And in all the disorientation of the fever, the feeling of being heckled, and the nervousness of directly talking to Him in the first place, time, for me, stood still. Sri Swamiji, in the hustle and commotion in the room, simply turned his head to someone I could not see and said loud enough for me to hear, "If she has enough respect to ask, I will have enough respect to answer," and silence fell on the room.

He started to offer me information about the Brotherhood, Speaking of Madam Blavinsky and others in their different incarnated and original names. But between my fever, his accent and my brief and simple knowledge of how this collective of souls work, I barely understood a word he said. The only sentence I remember him saying was "All of this information is in the Akashic Records, which is found in Tibet, but not on this dimension in Tibet, so there is no use going there, you won't find it."

After that, we sat in his presence for an hour and a half. A miracle of the day was that although still groggy, weak and a poster child for botox gone wrong, both Sarah and I walked out with our fevers gone and able to hold down some food. The real miracle of the bees though, was yet to 'bee' revealed.

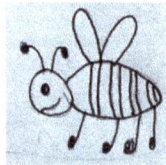

Narayana's Bee, aged 8

At the end of "the trip with the bees" I finally had the courage to ask for a one-on-one meeting with Paramahansa Satyasangananda Saraswati, affectionately known as Sw Satsangi.

It was this incredible woman, at the request and guidance of Sri Swamiji, that had found and acquired the land that we now know as Rikhiapeeth Ashram. She has been bestowed the title of Peethadhishwari of "Rikhia", holding the seat of honour and responsibility to uphold and embody the mandates of *Serve, Love and Give* as a living example to all. To me, she is the perfect embodiment of no mess, tell it like it is, utterly loving, compassionate and encouraging, with a hint of childlike playfulness that results in a laugh that coaxes flowers to bloom.

There is a tangible light that hits you as soon as her mind focuses on your being, at least, this is my experience. But when light shines on a personality, an ego, then shadow also rises to be seen, as it did on this day, resulting in a near panic attack of insecurity at being informed that my request had been granted. I got ten minutes of warning before our meeting, and that ten minutes was a whirl wind of "Oh my god, she's going to rip me to pieces, she knows I'm a complete fraud, she's going to tell me I'm full of ..." well not that I think she would use those terms, she wouldn't need to, I would get the message in more subtle ways. But as often with the insecure ego, it latches on to worst-case scenario and projects it forward, rather than sitting in the unknown. And like most worst-case scenarios, it was all in my head.

There is a teaching that I have heard many a veteran Swami lovingly whisper to people newer to the path and to the dynamics of having Guru guide your life. It goes something along the lines of: *At the foot of Guru, don't try and hide anything! It is better to be an honest imbecile in front of them, better to bare your soul without reserve, don't try to hide your faults and insecurities with a facade like you've got anything together. They see you and know you on levels we can't even comprehend. So better to be humbly and fallibly your idiotic self, than try and pretend you're something you're not.* An honest imbecile. I can do that!

I was ushered into her meeting room and was met with such a perfect example of a woman in power. Confidant and joyful but not loud or attention seeking. She was a blinding beacon of humility and kindness that in that moment no great shadow in me could spring forth, instead, intense gratitude, a teaspoon of bashfulness and only a dash of idiot bubbled forth from me. As I was being shown where to sit she sat on her chair calmly in silence.

wriggle wriggle fidget adjust...

"Um, I don't know the polite protocol for this, do you start? Do I start? Um..." I offered almost holding my breath not wanting even this to be the wrong thing to do or say.

"Let's start together," she said with a smile. Exhale... I think I'm in love.

We, well I, chatted about my life, about my work. As it is customary to request permission, or blessings from your Guru, once surrendered, (even though my commitment was not through a outward, formal initiation of Poorna Sannyas my internal pledge of surrender to Sri Swamiji was sincere) when embarking on any life altering decisions, I asked if it was in the highest and for blessings to marry the man, now initiated as Paramjyoti, that I had been seeing back in Vancouver, whom I had met shortly after I returned from my prayer and promise trip. She said it was and I decided to push my luck and ask if I could try and have a child with him. She said I could if I wanted, but not to come to the Ashram the next year if I was pregnant, to come after the child was born. Then I told her about this recurring dream/aspiration/hope to "build a retreat centre" Somewhere that people could come and reconnect to their hearts, to learn to live a Yogic lifestyle, to reconnect to nature. I could see it in the forest, but beyond that I had no idea. I put forth both boots of humility and exclaimed that if it was my Dharma I would put everything I had into it, if it was my ego I would drop it like a hot cake and pursue whatever she felt was right. I admitted that I was too ignorant to know the difference and I was hoping she would help me discern the direction.

Closing her eyes for a second or two she seemed to be listening to a far off trickle of sound, then coming back to this world she exclaimed "Yes, You should do it, but it won't be easy."

What in life that has true, soul permeating value is ever 'easy'?

"Where do you want to build this?" she asked.
"I have no idea, maybe Mt. Shasta?" I answered.
"No, Don't go where you will need to uproot yourself again"
"Um, can I go home to New Zealand?"
"No, there is already places you speak of there, where do you live again?"
"Vancouver BC, Canada"
"What's 12 hours inland from there?"
"I have no idea, maybe the Rocky Mountains?"
"Go there, and you will see where you need to be."

And like that, our first meeting was over.

Three days later, as I put my feet on North American soil my world went on fast forward. Within a week my beloved proposed marriage to me. Ten days later, on the first day of my first ovulation after returning from India, we conceived.

Astonished, and baffled, I called one of my shamanic teachers to deliver the news. Knowing of my previous diagnosis and my lack of being able to conceive before India she was delighted to say, "It's the bees!"

Confused I asked her to explain what she meant. She said that BVT, Bee Venom Therapy, is used as an anti-inflammatory for rheumatoid arthritis and multiple sclerosis, and is also the totem of fertility.

For years I had been trying to work at balancing the excess fire in my system and mind. I could see how it could take 80 bee stings in one hit to balance my fire, and bring by body into the frequency of fertility.

My prayer for a child was answered through a blessing from the bees.

We named our son Narayana, another name for Vishnu who is the God of the bees. With "maadhu" for a middle name, meaning "sweet like honey" to acknowledge and honour the Divine blessings of Sri Swamiji that brought him to us.

The Beloved's Arrival

> *Life's deepest knowing,*
> *Is delivered through,*
> *Sunflower Eyes,*
> *Divinities gift stands before me,*
> *No council sought,*
> *For no doubt dampens my joy,*
> *The water of life runs clear,*
> *For the time now is to drink,*
> *No longer looking for obstructions,*
> *Ways of potential escape,*
> *I lay my head beside you now,*
> *And bask in loves sweet nape.*
>
> S. H 2008

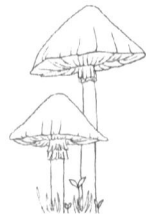

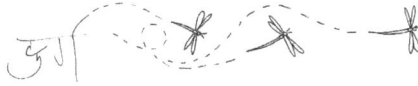

SEVEN

- Maha Samadhi and the Dream

A boon is a blessing directly from the Divine. A super power that mortals thirst for and the enlightened run from. These magical abilities are seen as distractions from the true goal, God realization, the true masters only utilize them in the service to humanity. Selflessly, never for personal gain.

One of Sri Swamiji's boons that was gifted to him was the ability to consciously choose the moment that his soul would leave his mortal frame. In true form, even in this moment, he chose the time that was most optimal, not for him, for the stars aligned were a tricky road to navigate, but for being able to makes use of a 'return ticket'. Being able to return to a human body as soon as possible and continue his work of uplifting humanity.

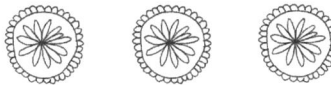

We were in New Zealand at this chosen moment in time, staying with my Mother and Stepfather. New Zealand in December is warm and bright, accelerating full speed towards the holiday season. Having only been there for a day or two I was changing Narayana's diaper, who was just seven weeks old, in the morning light of the sunroom. I was in a haze between absolute exhaustion being a new mum and feeling hung over from travelling from the other side of the world. Nevertheless, as you do when you have a small babe, I was in full swing, engaged in our goofy post diaper play time, cooing and cawing, doing whatever it took to invoke a smile on his face. Functioning moment to moment only to see his smile, to feel his little lungs rise and fall on my chest, his little fingers wrap around mine.

While we were engaged in our antics his eyes locked on mine. In this moment I experienced a wrinkle in the flow of time, a blip in the matrix, as a loving, kind voice, a mental frequency, other than my own, flashed through my head, "He's left his body." I looked at Narayana who was holding his eye contact with an otherworldly serious look on his face.

"He's left his body."

'You're crazy! It's sleep deprivation, it's the hormones, you're making stuff up!' all flashed through my mind in an instant. But as I looked at Narayana again, his eyes still looking at me, the same message flashed through me once more. "He's left his body," reverberated through my awareness with a clarity that I was not used to. My seven week old son was communicating with me telepathically. My mind started running with the dread that someone had died, I got up and started walking around the house. Paramjyoti was alive and well and my Stepfather was in the office doing accounting. I went back to crazy new mama drama, and let it go.

Within an hour, I was getting emails and Facebook messages that Sri Swamiji had left his body. It was not so much grief that over took me, after all, physically I had only been in his presence a few times and had only directly spoken to him once; yet my first response was an oscillation between, nothing has changed, and everything has changed. The tears came however, when I realized that, on this plane of existence, I would never get the opportunity to bring him our son and physically acknowledge to him that I was now a mother because of his intervention, blessing and Grace.

It was said to me sometime later that when a Master goes through any kind of initiation, or consciously leaves his or her body, that the surge forward of their consciousness has a similar affect as the moon does on the tides. As they step forward, all that are connected with them at the heart also steps forward, or has the opportunity to do so, evolving their own current level of awareness.

You see, about six months before, when I was five months pregnant with this bright light of a soul, I was diagnosed with Thyroid Cancer on the right side of my throat. Yogically, we are aware of the connections of the dimensional portals between what we call Swadhisthana, and Vishuddhi Chakras, which physically influence the uterus and throat respectively. What is happening in one chakra, is being mirrored in the other chakra. So when you have a bright light in your lower abdomen, as it shines on the wall of identified ego and karmas, it can surface undigested karma, or a dark shadow in the throat. The brighter the light, the darker the shadow. When there ceases to be a wall, individual personality or ego, or at least it becomes translucent, light and dark are no longer experienced with such harsh dualism. If there is no light, there is no dark. There just, is.

Through working with my teacher, Anandashakti, and within my own intuitive body, I could feel that the karma asking to be cleared at that time was a family karma and connected to the masculine, because it was the right side of the thyroid. This left the seeking to do with my dynamic with the masculine through my Father or Husband as I had no brothers. Seeing that Paramjyoti had also come through as a gift from the Divine I tried to focus on my understanding and patterning with my earthly Father who lived in Australia, with whom I had always been estranged. It was clear to me that our unborn son did not want to take on the identification of whatever truth/lie samskara or impression associated with Vishuddhi Chakra that was coming to the surface.

So it should have been no surprise that only 12 hours before Sri Swamiji left his body, my mother had broken down in tears and exclaimed that my father in Australia, was not my father at all. That I had grown up identifying with, and relating to a lie for the past 30 years. A lie that created a reality born out of fear, guilt and shame. This, was the manifestation of lies of the masculine that Narayana was not willing to take on upon his entry to the world. This was the gift of truth, associated with Vishuddi chakra, that I believe Sri Swamiji karmically gifted me as he left his body so that I would finally be able to step forward in my life being able to orientate a healthy and truthful relationship to the Divine Masculine, and would be able to unravel my feelings of mistrust of the Divine Feminine. After-all, it is taught that the first experience of trust a child has with it's first Guru, it's mother, is that she tells the child who his/her father is.

We are not victims to our earthly stories. Our human experience with other humans is but the leela, or play of the Divine to help us learn, heal and transcend the ignorance *we* have identified with as souls. So while on a human level I could look at this as a gross injustice towards me, that perspective would only perpetuate the hurt and mistrust of the cycle I was already in. To evolve, one has to be willing to recognize and experience, yet not identify with, the pain of the human experience. My human family, like all human families, are souls playing out the perfection of their karma, to give themselves and myself the opportunity to play out the perfection of our karmas. How I respond has more to do with what is inside me, and less to do with the external circumstances. I realized instead of pushing my Mother and biological father away out of hurt, I, for my own evolution, needed to learn quickly to forgive, to understand and to bring them closer in Love, and to consciously create opportunities for a relationship that is founded on honesty, sincerity and trustworthiness. It's a process, one that takes as long as it needs to, but this is the opportunity I was shown and encouraged energetically to do by Sri Swamiji's gift.

I believe that as a parting gift he gave all of us the perfect little karmic nudge, an opportunity to move through ignorance on a level that may have taken us years, even lifetimes, to do. That even his passing became a gift to all that were connected with him on the heart level. Mine, was the gift of Truth.

Layers of emotions surged through me as the days and weeks followed. Ultimately sinking into a "what now" feeling. I could feel that I had a connection with him on other, indescribable levels, but the only level my mind would fully trust was the tangible physical realm. It was then, amidst my despair, I had a dream that gave comfort, direction and courage to keep going.

In my dream, Sw Satsangi was standing in a non-descript place, with Paramjyoti and myself flanking her on her right and left sides respectively. She was holding both of our hands and I was balancing Narayana on my left hip. As we stood there, Sw Satsangi uttered a mantra, I have no idea what that mantra was but its effect was that it changed the dimensional perception of all of us and suddenly Sri Swamiji was standing in front of us. He looked at us and said, "Follow her, she will bring you to me." and then I woke up.

I held this dream close to my heart until a year later when I finally had the blessings of being in Sw Satsangi's physical presence again. I told her of the dream, and then asked, "So, will you? Will you take me to him? I think that means you're my in-body Guru now. Does it?" She was listening attentively, and as always, I could tell, with one ear listening to the intangible wisdom in the ether, she looked up and over, and with an air of it's not a big deal, matched with a slight smile and glint in her eye she simply said, "Yes."

And so, once again I dove into creating a relationship of complete trust and surrender with Sw. Satsangi as an embodiment of the Divine Mother. Trusting that through her, she would show me, guide me, and ultimately help me experience the beauty of the

Divine Mother and the Divine Father. And by opening to her guidance I will learn to attune to and follow the inner Guru.

"Lord Ram gave Hanuman a quizzical look and said, "What are you, a monkey or a man?" Hanuman bowed his head reverently, folded his hands and said, "When I do not know who I am, I serve You and when I Do know who I am, You and I, are One." -

Tulasidas

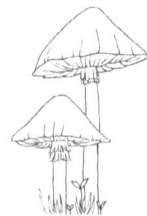

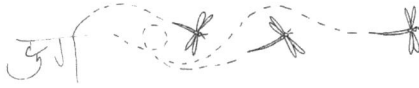

EIGHT

- This Is How God Speaks

"We all walk in mysteries. We do not know what is stirring in the atmosphere that surrounds us, nor how it is connected with our own spirit. So much is certain — that at times we can put out feelers of our soul beyond its bodily limits; and a presentiment, an actual insight is accorded to it: " Goethe.[17]

There are Divine messages all around us. Guiding and nudging and pointing us in the direction that is in our most high at that time. The trouble is, we have atrophied our heart intelligence, and it is this muscle that sees, connects to, and interprets these whispers as the openings to life's innate magic that they are. It is in this state that the paradigm of our reality can shift and we can perceive and receive finer threads of frequency, guidance and blessings. Steven Buhner calls this experience "following the golden threads."

"Golden threads always lead to a shift in perception, a traveling from one state of mind to another   We live in, are immersed within, a world of meanings not objects. But because the condensation of meaning occurs almost immediately when we see a physical object, none of us notice the process happening. It is so automatic we miss ourselves doing it."[18]

This meaning, this feeling, or heart intelligence, when we consciously interact with an aspect of our mundane sensorial stimulation, such as Mantra or the spontaneous interaction with a

---

[17] - from a letter written July 23rd 1820, quoted by Buhner, in The secret teachings of Plants.

[18] Buhner, Plant Intelligence and the Imaginal Realm

wild animal, is the tasseled end of a Golden Thread of frequency. When this tassel is followed, not just into the intellectual learning through references e.g. pictures or books, but into the heart's intelligence, you feel your way into perceptions of patterns and their meanings can spontaneously arrive at an experiential awareness of an expanded reality. This process gives us the tools and momentum to follow this shift of perception all the way to a leap of faith over the chasm of the unconscious, and into direct experience, into a reality that is multi dimensional, nuanced, and perfection in its objective, to using the illusion of duality to create the longing for a Re-membering of our true, innate Indigenous Nature.

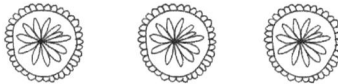

At five months pregnant we decided to take a road trip inland to look at land and generally see what in fact was twelve hours inland from Vancouver. I had never been to the interior of British Columbia or the surrounding area of Western Alberta and the solidity of the mountains, the clarity of the lakes and the friendliness of the people were all very appealing. We did a loop from Golden to Lake Louise, to Radium and back up to Golden. We looked at land, but with a lack of funds, we had to look for bare land. Buying bare land in BC is tricky in that you have to have a large deposit. It was a catch 22 that was exhausting to me and my belly. The energy of the area though was strained, forced and nothing seemed to quite line up. We returned home happy to have started the process, but feeling a little dejected about not knowing how it could possibly all come together.

And then life took over... Paramjyoti finished his nursing degree, I moved through cancer, we got married, Narayana was born. The city seemed to be suffocating me, and yet, somehow we got side tracked into buying an apartment in Vancouver. I like to think that we had some negative karma that had to play out before we could start fully on the main event. At least that is what I tell myself.

Anyone who has ever gotten to know me well, knows that Trust and Surrender are my biggest teachers. You could, read between the lines there and see that my biggest challenges are fear and control, alas, we send energy in to what we want to step towards, rather than what we need to step away from.

Time ticked on, and the pressure in me started to build. Two years after Sw Satsangiji[19] had suggested we find land and start a centre 12 hours inland from Vancouver and I was still sitting by Granville Island, waiting, waiting, and getting feverishly impatient. So much so, that one day I decided to pick an argument with those unseen and rummaged through an old box to find a pendulum. I got out a map of British Columbia and kindly demanded a reprieve from the pressure cooker of my impatient mind. Scanning the map to see if there was more energy "circling" one spot over another I moved up and down the Columbia Valley, situated 12 hours inland. Getting no clear guidance I somewhat haphazardly biffed the pendulum at the map. Out of desperation I looked at where it landed; right on Cranbrook, BC, a place that I now know is called ʔaq'am to the Ktunaxa people. Grabbing the computer I looked up the closest airport, only 20 minutes from the town, then looked up the size of the hospital, for after-all, Paramjyoti was going to need a job as a nurse to help us through, and turns out it was the Regional Hospital, the largest in the region.

We decided to go on an overnight trip and similarly scanned photos of real estate agents based in Cranbrook until we found one that resonated. Steve, the chosen real estate agent, picked us up

---

[19] Ji, is used at the end of a name to denote respect

from the airport and had an itinerary of four or five places around a one hour radius from Cranbrook for us to check out.

We loaded up our nine month old son in Steve's car and asked first to be taken to Moyie Lake. The reason for this was that waters are portals into this reality. I had made four medicine bundles of gratitude to be offered to the land and the waters asking for them to speak to us and guide us into the most high. Standing on the waters edge we opened up the four directions and asked to be shown clearly. We hopped back in the car and turned onto the highway. A moose stood just six feet off the road to which Steve exclaimed, "Whoa! I've been here six years and that's only the second moose I have ever seen. You have been here 30 minutes…" We looked up the medicine of the moose, "Sacred space has been opened," it read. We knew we were on the right track.

The truth is that the Divine is always communicating with us. The Divine mother's voice had come through the Earth herself. She's always whispering to us in the trees, the weather, the waters. Speaking and reaching out to our souls in language that our ears cannot hear. It's a language that needs the heart interpretation, a juggling between knowledge and feeling, intuition and discernment. Her language is our Mother Tongue. It's the most important communications we can listen to. Each communication has the opportunity to be medicine on a cellular level, a soul level. The intensity of her voice has the power to Re-member our fragmentations. Re-stitch the bridge between head and heart rendering us reconnected, awake and aware of our wholeness once more. Embodying her words is our reason for living. To hear her words, to fully understand them, to embody them and to share them with others. Giving birth to the Mother's Song is played out on every level of creation, including our own.

When I enquire to the medicine of a particular animal or bird I always take into account where I am experiencing it. If I am in New Zealand I look to the local indigenous interpretation. If I am at home in the Purcell Mountains, I look to the local Ktunaxa belief, or at least the "Native American" stance. If I am in India, I search the understanding from there. I try to submerge my soul into the Land's frequency wherever I am, rather than trying to impose my belief system onto it.

The first property was down in Yahk. Between the cigarette butts on the ground and the guns on the wall, the energy of the land that hosted the little hunter's cabin was suffocated in grief and I could hardly breathe. Next was Bull River, where we ran around for 30 mins looking for the property stakes to see where the boundaries were. Frustration and anger rose in me, this was not a good sign, so we kept going. After another couple of properties that didn't feel right I was again disheartened. Narayana was grumpy from being in the car all day, Paramjyoti was, well, Paramjyoti, quietly looking sideways at me wondering who was going to blow a fuse first. We decided to drive up to Kimberley where one of our student's parents had granted us a bed for the night, but as we wound our way up to the little mountain town, Steve said he wanted to show us something. It was not a property for sale, but something he thought we would like to see.

We turned down St. Mary's Valley and for 30 minutes we drove down a winding dirt road sandwiched between a sheer cliff of rock and a river. My city mind took over and I started to question Steve's intentions for driving us so far away from civilization. Just before a bridge, Steve pulled off the road and stopped a few feet from the water. It had just started to drizzle, but with one medicine bundle left, I wanted to offer it to this beautiful valley. As I unlatched Narayana's seat belt I glanced at Paramjyoti's face. His eyes had gone wide as he said, "Look!" Certain there was a bear or cougar behind me my nervous system went into fight or flight, but obediently I turned around. There, we found ourselves engulfed in a blanket of golden light. So encompassing that we could not even see the hillside right in front of us. Each droplet of rain was catching the sun right at the perfect angle, creating an otherworldly experience. All three adults just stood there, mouths agape watching the fairy like sparkles dance around us. I grabbed the medicine bundle and walked down to the river. Uttering a prayer to the spirits of the valley, asking that they receive this humble token of our gratitude, I said I would Light Weave for the waters set the intention that my offering be used in whatever way the Spirits of the land would think was the most high. I toned one long note, then another, and another, and as I changed my frequency of sound, the rain changed frequency of precipitation. From a drizzle, to rain, to pouring, and back to rain, absolutely in time with my singing. I would think I was imagining this, but Steve, a man we had only met that morning was standing on the bank yelling, "Who are you? And what are you doing?????" "I don't know!" I yelled through the rain, "I'm not doing anything!" and I ran back to the car to get out of the rain.

As we drove out of the valley we were stopped by a family of three mountain goats, a mum, dad and kid. Patiently we waited for them to get off the road, thinking they would drop down towards the river and pasture, the path of least effort, but instead they turned and started the hard, steep and laborious trek up the shale rock cliff on our left, showing us directly their medicine of stepping forward confident in their footing; walking uncommon paths and going to heights not many others would attempt. As we drove past them, a double rainbow arched over the road landing in the St. Mary's Lake on our right.

The next month we went back to India and were gifted the opportunity to tell Sw Satsangi of these experiences directly. We relayed each detail to her like children explaining the wonder of seeing a shooting star for the first time. Her response, "THIS is how God speaks, this is what you follow, move there and integrate into the community. Look for land, and build the Centre."

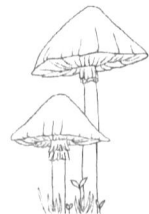

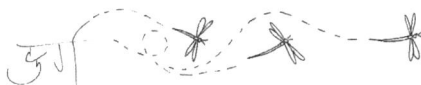

NINE

- Wake Up, Surrender, Receive

Come,
Let us listen,
To the whispers suspended between the here and now
The ones we will only fully understand,
In the silence of tomorrow.

We love to think that all our Asana and Pranayama, techniques and tricks are getting us closer to the prize of happiness, peace, health, enlightenment. Consistent and dedicated practice of these actions do make a difference, don't get me wrong, but to me, they are the individual actions we do to humbly prepare for Grace. To build up the muscle of awareness, of Re-membrance, requires a deep listening to the hearts whispers, reconnecting our frayed nervous systems, shifting our understanding, our perception of this human experience until we can recognize the song of Love and dance each day with the Divine as the DJ. It's not the romantic love between two people, the Love that is the song of the Divine permeates the whole of creation; Atma, weaving golden threads of interconnection between each tree, animal, building, person. We like to think we are evolving because of our own efforts, but experiences of Grace, or shifts of consciousness, in my life, have been completely spontaneous, Divinely gifted, absolutely nothing directly to do with my will, intention, or mundane efforts.

One time, while in India, I was sleeping in the same room as Paramjyoti and Narayana, who was two years old at the time. I woke in the morning in a completely different state of awareness than I had ever experienced before. The sensation that I awoke to is hard to put into words, for it simply does not translate to experience, but there was a frequency running through me that was otherworldly, and yet, not separate from the mundane world. I was clear, calm, no random thoughts running through my mind bar the "whoa, what is happening" enquiries, and yet every level of my being was running an octave higher than it usually did. I decided that the best thing to do was to try and absorb as much of this frequency as possible and go back to sleep. I asked Paramjyoti to take Narayana for the morning, thinking I would wake in an hour back to "normal".

Alas, when I woke up 2.5 hours later, I was still very much bathed in the same frequency. No longer tired, I got up and started getting ready for my day. Again, I thought that moving around and engaging with life would shift my perspective, but it didn't. The frequency running through me only enhanced my experience. So I tidied our room, cleaned the bathroom, organized our clothes. Tasks I don't often relish were done with overwhelming joy and simplicity. No thought crossed my mind that was not completely present to the task at hand. "Is this a minuscule taste of reality that is the constant experience of the Masters? What would it be like to move through my reality with this as my base frequency all the time? What would that look like?" Deciding to just be grateful I spent the morning alone, in silence and busy in mundane actions of folding clothes, making beds etc.

By mid morning I thought Paramjyoti might be going a little crazy with our toddler, I reluctantly walked over to the main compound. Intuitively knowing that as soon as I started to talk to people my experience of this frequency would subside, which it did.

I wanted to talk to Sw Satsangi about the experience, to seek an explanation, or a labeling I could hold on to, that I could give it for future reference, but she was not seen for the day before my experience or the two days after. Finally, a week or so later, I had the chance to mention it to her. I asked if she thought it had anything to do with whatever she was doing in her absence from the public eye. That maybe my soul was sensitive to a particular sadhana she was engaged in that perhaps had permeated the ashram. Her response was the playful inconclusive half smile, and slight shrug she gets when she wants me to stop talking. I took that as a cue just be grateful to the Divine for the gift of experience. And if you're wondering, no, I have not had the experience since. God willing, some day.

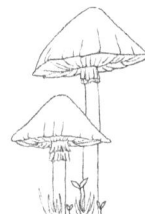

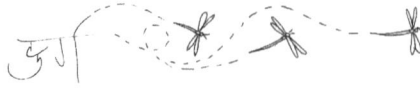

TEN

- The Boon OF Vak

Anxiety is something many would describe as a burden they bare on a daily, sometimes constant basis. For them, it is, "the song that never ends, it just goes on and on my friend," (you started singing it didn't you?). Anxiety is contagious like that, an epidemic in our society. Some would say they 'suffer' from it. An anxious mind is untethered to the Light, ungraspable thoughts flapping wildly over the dark and bottomless chasm of the unknown tomorrow. Anxiety, as fears spawn, is what we interact with when we don't have the courage to look directly in fear's face and ask it what the hell it's so afraid of?

But what if we, as a society, have anxiety all wrong? Like pain, what if anxiety is the misunderstood villain we are taught from knee high to shun at all costs, and have yet to question? What if that shot of anxiety that flashes through your brain, was nothing but an internal alarm clock going off to remind you to pray? To trust, to call out to your Ishtadevata[20], to surrender to Thy will. What if it was a cadenced song of Re-membrance to acknowledge that you are not in control, and that this moment, by Re-membering to anchor into trust, is an opportunity to open to love on a level you have not yet dared to entertain?

What if anxiety was your temple's call to announce it's time to plant seeds of Divine Trust in your heart so the flowers of Surrender will have their day of blossoming?

---

[20] Ishtadevata: Is your personal form of the Divine that is most inline with your highest potential in this lifetime.

You see Trust, in the Divine, is the seed of our Indigenous Nature and when planted in the depth of our beings, beyond the reach of anything worldly, sprouts the innately joyful awareness of our interconnectedness with all beings, seen and unseen. This awareness of interconnection through the veins of empathy is incredibly powerful and blooms forth the sweetly scented flowers of Surrender and Service. For once this interconnection is experienced, you recognize that the suffering in others, is in fact nothing but the reflection of your own despair unsung. By directing our own life-force energy towards relieving the 'other' is in fact, through our interconnectivity, applying a soothing balm to our own soul. It is the human expression of Poornamadah[21].

From these sweet flowers of Surrender and Service, basks a scent of contentment that permeates the fabric enclosing the bosom of Love. From the dimensional foundation of Love, germinates the new sprout of Truth which takes all of the DNA and Re-membrance of each stage of awareness and growth from the previous incarnations and blooms forth a new flower. This flower is so complete, so refined that it only needs two petals, which are lovingly referred to as Sun and Moon, Ha and Tha[22], knowing that that which lies between them is "everything" reduced to a single bindu, a point, a seed of Yog - Union.

When we look at a complete plant, we can see how even though different parts of the plant look different, for example: leaf and flower, how they act differently, and have different destinies and roles, there is no doubt that for one part to fulfill its destiny the other parts have to be fulfilling theirs. Their interconnectivity is fait accompli for it has all manifested from the same seed. All the different aspects, shapes, sizes, roles and abilities, although may be

---

[21] Poornamadah: The understanding that all comes from the whole, and nothing can ever be added nor subtracted from that. All coming and going of life is but perception.

[22] Ha - Sun Tha - Moon - the two words that make up "Hatha Yoga"

varying from one part of the plant to the next, are part of one organism. And so are we. When we tap into seed consciousness and stop identifying with being a leaf or a flower and our personal role, and instead take an interest in how we can support any aspect of the plant to thrive, we are able to communicate and guide any part of the plant. How? Through the portal frequencies of water, and vibration.

When someone is functioning from an expanded awareness of their role and potential while simultaneously aware of their interconnectivity with all beings, one realizes that the fluidity and purity of the emotions, e-motion: energy in motion, that you float on, gives buoyancy to the words you speak, your manifested vibration, and are the very threads that weave our reality. This allows one to utilize the power of your words to direct the waters of reality into a direction that is in the most high, just like the moon pulls the tides.

This ability to use speech to support and guide manifestation in this way is called Vak Siddhi and is a boon that is said comes from the awakening of Vishuddhi Chakra. The ability to manifest whatever you speak can of course be very dangerous for anyone who has not yet purified the mind to a point of not being at the whim of random or irrational thoughts. For what you think, you focus on, what you focus on, you are likely to speak about, what you speak about, you create.

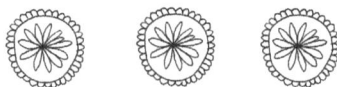

This I have witnessed directly through the guidance of Sw Satsangi. You see, two years after the golden veils of light and rain changing frequency, after we moved to Kimberley BC to look for land, we were still no closer to stepping forward. In fact, we were painfully stuck in the grips of real estate karma back in Vancouver, owning an apartment there that did not hold its value after we purchased it.

That first year we were challenged to pay rent for a home in Kimberley and a mortgage in Vancouver on a single family income, stressed to the max at not finding the land and not having the cash flow to do it either. Finally, we managed to rent out the apartment but it was a band aid on a wound of responsibility. It was, looking back, one of the most challenging times in our family to date.

Humbly, we sat in front of Sw Satsangi and explained to her that we were no closer to finding land and were at a loss with this apartment in Vancouver that was creating levels of stress that were debilitating.

The ego wants the concerned look, the hand holding and the leaning forward as you are imparted a secret. But in reality, our issues that create us so much stress are really the result of identifying as doers in our little personal ego sit-com called life. Masters, such as She, are aware of a much bigger picture and rightfully, seem to look at us the same way I would look at a one year old who wants another slice of cheese but can't have it. The fact that she even entertains a meeting with us, so that we can babble our worldly problems to her is an immeasurable act of compassion, kindness and utter patience. So, her response can almost seem at times flippant, a brushing off of instructions that seem inconsequential. I imagine if you are not in the right frame of mind, you could almost miss them. Brushing them off as mere polite conversation. But to me, each word that she utters is a blessing, a gift that is not to be discarded because of the wrapping. Each thing she says to us, although on the surface seems easy and almost trivial, is but a fleck of paint off a mansion of exquisite architecture.

As she adjusts her seat and throws her dhoti[23] over her shoulder, she advises us to, "Go home, sell your apartment.

---

23 Dhoti: A rectangular piece of unstitched cloth worn by a renunciate.

Paramjyoti go back to casual nursing and buy land. Don't teach while you build, just focus on building. Oh and you don't have enough money to buy land, so you will have to lease until you can purchase it." My first reaction was fear, as my little ego started to inwardly yabber, 'ah, you are either enlightened or you're crazy!, cause you don't understand, the market in Vancouver has gone down blah blah blah...' Shivani. You asked, she has spoken. Trust and follow her instructions.

A few short months later back in the majestic mountains of BC, we found ourselves in the throws of the Navaratri Sadhana, the 9 Nights of Durga. It involves 5am recitations of the Sundaraya Lahari, that are a gorgeous sadhana praising and invoking the blessings of the Divine mother, that I simultaneously look forward to and dread, thoroughly enjoy once there but still sometimes I wish I could participate from a couch with a coffee in my pajamas. Our tenants who had been renting the apartment for less than a year had gotten pregnant and had decided to go back to Ontario to live. My stomach hit the floor as they let us know they were moving out. My nervous system bolted for the gate like a horse trained to run at the sound of a gun. So habitual is my anxiety that to counter balance its chokehold on me I started to carry around a photo of Sri Swamiji, to focus on surrender, trust and non doer-ship through the experience. Every time I thought about how we were going to sell a one bedroom apartment in Vancouver, when 130 of them were not selling. I was rendered continuously nauseous. With every nauseous wave of dread over me I would pull out the picture from my pocket and mutter incoherently, "This is your apartment Sri Swamiji, your bills, your problem. I lay it at your feet... let thy will be done."

The middle day of our Navaratri Sadhana is dedicated to Laxmi, the mother in the form of abundance and virtue. We had placed the apartment on the market just two days earlier and on this particularly cold Wednesday in April I had made it to the supermarket in the slushy snow. As I walked into the supermarket my phone rang. It was the real estate agent. My nervous system did that flip, drop, queasy dance as I answered. She informed me that through some unexplainable circumstances her website had been found up on another agents computer when the agent arrived at his office on the Monday morning. This particular agent was trying to help his cousin and his cousins' fiancé, who was from West Bengal of India, to buy a place. They instantly loved ours and our agent had already received a written offer with the full amount that we figured the market would give us at that time!Not even three full days after putting it on the market! Pacing around the supermarket with the phone against my ear, zigzagging in and out of aisles with an empty cart, tears of relief streaming my face, I called Paramjyoti to let him know and to get his go ahead to accept the offer. He responded by telling me that he had gotten to work that morning and had promptly quit his full time line and had gone back to casual. Something we had not discussed as a couple and yet, in one morning two out of three of Sw Satsangi's instructions had manifested.

I spent the rest of the day floating from one task to the next, bubbling with the unburdened freedom only being relieved of an unwanted mortgage can give. I called my friend to tell her the good news and it sparked her to mention that the previous evening she had had dinner with a local couple who had land out at Ta Ta Creek that they were thinking of selling privately, for the right price, the right project, and to the right people. "You should give them a call," she said, "and see if you can check it out."

I hung up only to turn around and dial her friend Dave's number. We planned on meeting the next morning to go and walk the land. It was a blue bird day with a foot of snow on the ground. You couldn't drive all the way in for the road was not maintained in the winter.

As we hiked from one end of the property to the other, we chatted and trudged through the snow, up hill and over logs to a spot where a derelict camper was parked. It was the spot, he told us, that was the obvious building site on the property. Situated in the foothills of the Purcell Mountains, the views across the Columbia Valley to a panorama of the Rocky Mountains were exquisite. Not another living soul for miles, it was so quiet you could hear the squirrel's nails tap on the branches as they scurried to tell the news of the humans that had invaded!

As Narayana and Paramjyoti explored, Dave and I stood in the snow and chatted.

"So, do you like it?" he enquired.

"Well it's not really about whether or not I like it, it's not really even up to me, this endeavour is bigger than me, I'm just looking for a sign from Sri Swamiji, from the Divine. Something to tell us we are where we are destined to be," I replied.

"What kind of sign do you mean?"

"Well, I don't know," wondering how much of our woo woo existence I should divulge, "I'm looking for something, something like golden veils of light, or rain changing frequency," feeling bashful and slightly embarrassed. "But it's a blue sky day so I don't think that will be happening. Maybe, prints, or scat or something, something out of the ordinary for the Divine to tell us we are where we need to be."

"Like maybe an antler? This is an Elk corridor, and it is April, so they will be shedding soon."

"Yeah, maybe, but there is a foot of snow on the ground, and I can't see my feet let alone an antler on the ground."

I called out to Paramjyoti that we needed to find a sign from Sri Swamiji, from the Divine, to let us know if we were on the right path.

Before I could even shut my mouth from talking, Paramjyoti walked ten feet away, saw something white sticking an inch out of the white snow and put his hand down to see what it was. Birthed out of the snow, like the phoenix rising out of the fires he pulled up a seven-pointed Elk antler. Seven, the frequency of Yoga. Dave started to shriek with delight, like a dog who just saw a huge bone. "Oh my God! We have to find the other one! Oh my god! I have never seen one so big on this property, it's the sign! It's the sign! Ok! You can lease the land for two years and then you can purchase it once you have a cabin on the property, that way you can afford the down payment! Ok! We have to find the other one!"

While he started looking at nearby trees for signs of rubbing, I took a photo of Paramjyoti holding the antler and emailed it to Sw Satsangi to seek blessings and confirmation that this, indeed, was where we needed to be. And if it was, would she do us the honour of naming it, for I didn't want it to be

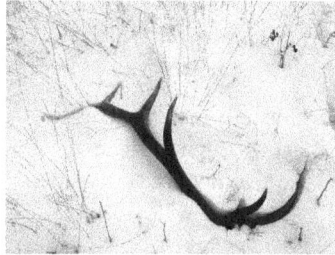

The infamous 7 pointed antler.

"our" place, I wanted it to be its own identity with its own destiny offered to the light bearers in gratitude. I could not venture into it, for diving into lawyers, and leases, and building on land we didn't own was yet another reason for my nervous system to flip flop with fear. If we were going to do this, we had to be fully rooted in Trust and Faith. It had to come *through us*, not from us.

Expecting to wait the usual two to three weeks for a official reply from the Ashram I started to look for the other antler as well, yet not 10 minutes later my phone beeped with a response from Sw Satsangi. "Yes. Step forth with the blessings of Guru. Its name is Ishtadev Niwas." Quickly I responded with, "Well then, who is the Ishtadev?" "Guru" was the reply. And the seed was planted, that this space was to be dedicated to Sri Swamiji himself. A home for him in the Rocky Mountains.

Ishtadev Niwas, Home of Supreme Bearers of Light.

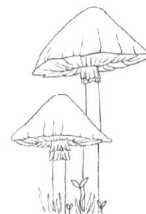

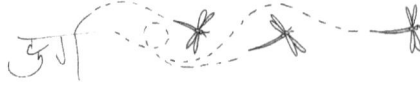

ELEVEN

- Foundational Moments

"It was not in the wild but in the veld where humans went to remember".[24] *Martin Prechtel*

"Niwas", as we lovingly call her, is a veld. A field or a piece of land that is in a buffer zone between "civilization" and "the wild". She is a place to come and Re-member our potential, to honour the Holy in Nature, the Divine as something that is not separate from ourselves, but a Self that we, are in fact, a part of. She has her own destiny, and we are her caretakers. Our role is to be in service to Her, Devi in her form of land, to help create space, and hold space so the Light, that Sri Swamiji embodied, has a place to touch down and touch the souls of all who come. A place where the Holy is fed, and all those that come can Re-member how to feed their souls, how to live integrated with the land, with the trees, and with the animals that reside on her, once again being part of a greater family. She has memory, that has lain dormant for many years, memory that is ready to be awakened, to be shared, and to be Re-membered into our own being. *For if one awakens, all that live in that house, too, shall wake.*

It is in this vein that we reside on her belly, and she resides in our heart. And the process of understanding this relationship, and role we play has been full of magical moments. Each one reminding us, that this place we call home, and all that it embodies, comes through us, not from us for the purpose of something, much greater than us alone.

---

[24] from the The Unlikely Peace at Cuchumaquic.

There is a yogic teaching, that we gain knowledge through learning, and we gain wisdom by applying experience to the knowledge. It makes life a little bit of a science experiment and enables us to focus on the process of life, rather than the outcomes.

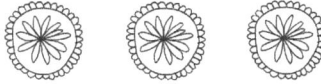

The summer of 2012 we pulled our 12 foot camper onto the land, with a husband working shift work, a two year old child, two dogs, a porta-loo and a dream. That summer was a daily opportunity of applying this teaching. I was simultaneously riddled with my ol' friend anxiety over money and the unknown, and ferociously needed to use this as the biggest opportunity to experience trust in the Divine, through the forms of Sri Swamiji and Sw Satsangi.

Shivani, being a favourable name for Shiva's wife has, for me, always been an embodiment of Durga - the fearless mother. Knowing this, faith and trust have been my biggest opportunities for growth. In other words I have been known to be completely chicken shit.

Action, speaking louder than words, the only way I could fathom to keep my alignment towards the light during the first months at Niwas was to perform a Satyananda Gayatri Havan[25] every morning to implore Sri Swamiji for his grace and support towards our endeavour. And he did.

A week or so in I had a Geru[26] coloured dragonfly land on my Geru coloured dhoti before the Havan at 6.30am and sit there for a good 20 mins. It was my sign that our efforts were being

---

[25] Havan: A Vedic fire ceremony.

[26] Geru: Traditionally the colour of the soil of the Ganga river is a rust colour or deep orange.

heeded not only by Sri Swamiji, but by the Divine mother as well. It is recognizing these signs that gives us courage to keep going.

The next few months we started to build Satyam Kutir, the main teaching house, dedicated to Sri Swamiji through this nickname while he was Sw Sivananda, Satyam. House of Truth.

The generosity of the local community was humbling.

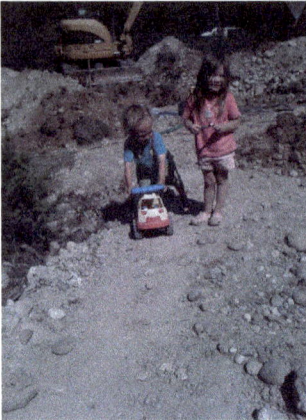

Narayana and Riley playing while we built Satyam Kutir

Shortly after acquiring the land a student gifted a sum of money to help start the building process. This was matched by local trades people who donated half their time, and were paid for the other half. These same trades people are fully hired today to help us continue the growth of the place. Local companies donated time to teach us the skills to build timber frames and straw bale walls. Other companies donated materials that were ends of lines or unable to be used for other projects.

It was truly an embodiment of the teaching: If you have the money to throw at it, it will be built on the foundation of money and will attract the people who are in it for the money. If you don't have the money, you will need to build it on the foundation of community, creativity and Grace. This is the foundation of Love. Places that are built on the foundation of Love stand the test of time.

The support of the community, to us, is the manifestation of the Grace and good will of the Guru's glance, it was a humbling experience of the power of community and the kindness of people wanting to bring beauty and good into the world.

August that year was one of the hottest on record. Days on end being over 30 degrees meant that in the three foot foundation of Satyam Kutir, it was regularly over 40 degrees with the reflection of the insulation heating up the rebar. Hanging the rebar stirrups was like playing the game Operation as a kid. The gap between them being too narrow for my shoes, I had to work barefoot and every time my ankle touched a piece of metal I got a small burn. It meant I had to work with extreme care, awareness, embrace ice cream and occasionally cry from exhaustion and frustration as the nails to hang the stirrups would warp under the heat and they would all fall like dominos along the 50ft wall.

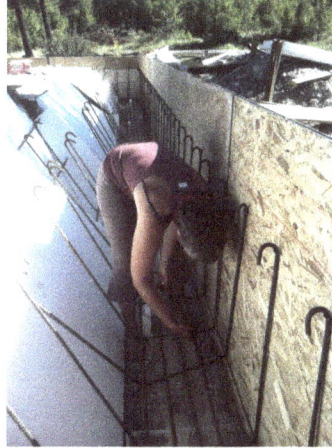

Hanging rebar stirrups
for Satyam Kutir

The night before we poured the concrete though was one I will never forget. It had been a challenging day of finishing off the prep work for the pour. Paramjyoti and I were both physically, emotionally and mentally exhausted and had been bickering all afternoon. They say if you want to see if your marriage will stand the test of time, build a house together. I now understand this saying acutely. In the evening we wanted to set an intention for the next day through a small ceremony of mantra and offerings. We placed rose quartz (for love), clear quartz (for Divine light), turquoise (as an honouring of the native connection to the land), ceremonial tobacco, sage, lavender, and a few other select offerings in each corner of the foundation, as well as a photo of Sri Swamiji circled in crystals in the middle of the building. We chanted to Ganesha to ask for blessings and the removing of obstacles and offered other chants and song to align the building with the highest intention we could. That it may be a house of Truth and Light for all who come.

When it was done we went to bed to prepare for the next day where I would welcome the concrete trucks and Paramjyoti would pull a 12 hour shift at the hospital.

That night though, something happened. I awoke, to a lucid dream/vision of sorts. Knowing my body was still in the camper asleep, my consciousness was roused by noises up by the foundation. As usual, I was afraid but willed my mind to creep up, hiding behind trees, to see what it was.

In my lucid dreaming/vision state, I saw a flying object, literally a UFO - unidentified flying object - come and hover over the space of the foundation. A beam of light came, shone down on to the space and beings "beamed" down onto the centre of what would be Satyam Kutir. I can't say for sure how many beings were there, but three of them stood to the side as the others did a Parikrama[27], A circumvention clockwise around the outside of the foundation. These three blew conches, large shells, and rang bells. Once the Parikarma was completed by everyone they all "beamed" back up into the ship of sorts, and disappeared.

I woke in the camper and bolted straight upright in bed. I knew then that our efforts had been heeded and that the foundation of Satyam Kutir had been blessed by beings of light. The foundation had been set, and we were ready to set it in stone.

---

[27] Parikrama, term used for walking around a sacred site clockwise.

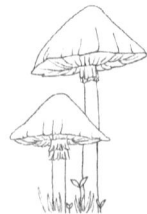

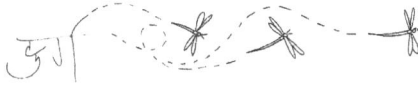

TWELVE

- The Onion of Indignation.

"Be patient toward all that is unsolved in your heart and try to love the questions themselves, like locked rooms and like books that are now written in a very foreign tongue. Do not now seek the answers, which cannot be given you because you would not be able to live them. And the point is, to live everything. Live the questions now. Perhaps you will then gradually, without noticing it, live along some distant day into the answer."
— *Rainer Maria Rilke*

So often in our reality, we try and change our external circumstances to support, or create a more pleasant internal experience. We want our surroundings to be the answer to an internal question we have not yet prepared ourselves to fully live into. And because we know what we want, but are not yet ready to change to become a being that can hold such responsibility as our wildest dreams manifested, we blame the outside world, create stories of how it's done us wrong and reject it. We then move onto a new place and expect it to be better. But we are still there, the same 'ol us, still not quite ready to live our answers, for fear of it being us that needs to change. And this is why I love the Ashram. For it is a container of light that doesn't need me to like it. It doesn't need me to be this, or be that, and yet it welcomes me with open arms and embraces me with opportunities to Re-member. The ashram is a bubble of light with a titanium casing. Creating a container for me to live into my own answers and understandings, while not budging if my ego wants to hit up against it. The ashram vibrates at such a frequency that it brings to the surface all that we are not, much like how our bodies will push to the surface a splinter embedded under our skin, so we can heal, Re-member and once again embody the essence of who and what we truly are.

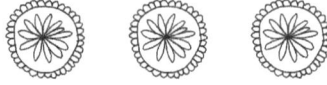

***

2013 offered the invitation and an opportunity to go to the Ashram in India for three months. This would be the longest stay I had ever done. I was excited, feeling that Rikhia was my true home. I was thrilled to go and immerse myself for longer than I had ever done. I had desires, fantasies - bordering expectations, to be brought into the fold as a temporary resident. At last, I was going to be included. Be on the "in". And of course, with all these high school samskaras of inclusion vs rejection bouncing around in my unconscious I was offered a wonderful opportunity to face, and let go of my need to be included in the way *I* expected. Upon arrival to the ashram, it was made clear, and quite rightly, that we were still temporary guests. Just ones that were there for longer than most.

My karma yoga during the beginning of that trip was in the kitchen. It was an easy place to have flexibility with Narayana being three years old. Needless to say, I spent the first six weeks chopping onions and crying. My ego went into a four year old tantrum. In hindsight, it was mildly embarrassing, and necessary. I wanted to sit with the big kids. I wanted to be taken seriously. I wanted to be acknowledged. I wanted, I wanted, I wanted... I needed, to go inside and see the blessing of being able to be there for three months in the first place. I needed, to soften into the opportunity of being a mother in the ashram - which is not for the faint of heart. Instead, I felt simultaneously entitled and rejected, even in the face of such kindness from some of the most senior swamis. We were offered so much personal attention, kindness and counseling by them, and yet all I saw were inconsistencies everywhere. My ignorant, limited mind and lack of information grabbed hold of each, seemingly external unfairness, it could. A karma sannyasin[28] that had come for four days to the ashram with her two year old was ushered to sit with the poorna sannyasins for Puja[29]. Narayana and I were asked to sit at the back with the guests. I screamed on the inside and cried on the outside.

One morning, as Paramjyoti and I were allowed to take alternate dates to go to morning Puja, allowing Narayana to sleep, I sat next to Sri Swamiji's Samadhi Sthal[30], the place where his physical body rests facing the morning sun as it dawns a new day, and a clear voice came through my mind, "Stop being so *indignant*."

Being that the English language has never been my strong point I asked a friend at breakfast what her understanding of "indignant" meant. She said her understanding of the word was "Being annoyed or angry at what is perceived as unfair treatment." Which when I later consulted a dictionary was pretty spot on, both in her understanding of the word and what I was feeling!

Sigh. I started to realize that this frequency and feeling of indignation was such a low-grade constant of my every day experience that I didn't even notice it half the time. I started to see that it tainted a tremendous amount of my reality in and outside of the Ashram. It was an aspect of my personality that was holding me away from Love, from the peace of this moment, and it was up to me to heal it. Yet, with most wounds, they offer a perspective that seems so justified that it is more of a process of peeling layers, much like onions, than a pill that makes the pain go away. The irony was

---

[28] Karma Sannyasin: Someone who is committed to the teachings of renunciation of attachment to material possessions and emotional ties, but still lives out in the world with household responsibilities.

[29] Puja: An act of worship

[30] Samadhi Stahl: Resting Place

not lost on me. Guru's ego-dectomy indeed has a sense of humour as its scalpel.

Six weeks into our three month stay we asked for permission to attend the 50 year Golden Jubilee of the Bihar School of Yoga. With Sw Satsangi's blessing we went, and arrived the morning that Amma, Swami Niranjanananda's mother, left her body. As we knew we were coming back to Rikhia we left our passports and personal belongings there, another symptom of wanting to belong and feel as though we were more than temporary, and were promptly advised that we needed them to be allowed into the Munger Ashram. After tension and begging, Grace prevailed, and they said we could stay but please remember for next time. Tired from our five hour trip by car to Munger we headed over to the office to find out where we were staying. As we waited for crowds to disperse Narayana forgot to tell us he needed to use the bathroom, NOW!, and promptly pooped on the front door step. Embarrassed is not really the word for my experience, mortified might be more accurate. There was no blame on Narayana, he was three and potty training. The blame was on us and being so distracted with the news of Amma's passing and the passport fiasco after a long drive, we had forgotten he didn't have a diaper on.

We got to our room, settled in and went to the Puja. The tantric Yoginis were performing a Sri Vidya Puja. Stunning and intense in every way. It was funny to watch them steal glimpses and little smiles at the little white three year old bouncing around in the aisle. He made googley eyes at them and waved, causing giggles from the Yogini's standing to the side. The love between them was positively tangible and soon, not so positively, so was my stomach. No sooner had the Puja finished, that I started to throw up. Ashrams in India are not easy places to be sick. Bathrooms are rarely easily accessible, and meals, even if all you are eating is plain rice to invoke some sort of energy, or at the least give you something to throw up, might as well be a mile away, the distance ensuring that you start walking 45 minutes early and take multiple breaks just to get there in one piece. After I started throwing up, Narayana started, then Paramjyoti. Narayana was convinced, and I must admit I tend to agree, that it was the power of the Sri Vidya Puja that the Tantric Yoginis were performing that sent us on a fast tract to full family purification. He has been simultaneously terrified and reverent of the Yoginis ever since.

While the boys were perking up within 24 hours, I on the other hand was convinced I would never look at food again. The rest of the stay in Bihar was a hobbled blur of chanting, puking and stairs. There were just - so - many - stairs.

Upon returning to Rikhia, Sw Satsangi asked how our time in Munger was. I sheepishly told her that we had all been sick, and that I, four days later, was still unable to hold anything down. A particular and endearing half smile crossed her face as she said that I indeed looked purified. Dreading my assumed return to the kitchen I asked her to give me something to focus on. A word, a teaching, a mantra, something I could demand my mind latch onto while I peeled and chopped onions on the outside while secretly dueling with my indignant demon on the inside. She said she would think about it and get back to me.

The next day, one of the Swamis had been told to find me and give me reassignment. I was to work on a project in the morning, and Paramjyoti was to look after Narayana. Then, in the afternoon I was on Mama duty, and Paramjyoti would help in the medical clinic. The project, I was informed, was to work on collating a book for publication. I was to research in the library articles and satsangs by either Sri Swamiji, or Sw Śivananda on the topics Serve, Love and Give. Then, I was to have full access to all the photos taken from the last five years and match them up to the articles, creating a book of inspiration. As the Swami's details were registered in my rational mind, my soul heard one message, "You get to sit in a room, by yourself, no interruptions, no child, and you get to read the words of Sri Swamiji and Sw Sivananda. Then, you get to look at every intimate photo of the last five years. You will see images and details of events like Sri Swamiji's Maha Samadhi and Sw Niranjan's Abhishek initiation into the Sannyas Tradition, as though you were there for every moment."

After six weeks of ego hell, this was soul heaven. Every satsang had a transmission, which my heart soaked up like the first rain after a drought. Motherhood had not allowed me a moment to even have an uninterrupted thought, let alone the opportunity to read. Heck, I hadn't even been to the bathroom alone in three years. This opportunity was such a balm to my soul, each photo was imprinted on my heart, each word enveloped by the marrow of my bones.

Sw Satsangi seemed to be pleased with my efforts towards this project, and on our next trip I was offered a copy as prasaad[31]. Sankalpa Of A Paramahansa. Of course the final product was, in part, different to how I had left the project. Gratefully, for my ego probably couldn't handle it if it wasn't. Still, the gift was not in the finished tangibility, but in the process of creation.

If every month I have spent in the ashram has taken me about six months to even start to digest and absorb the subtle differences and opportunities, then our three month trip has taken me years. I have never engaged with an onion since without checking in with where I am in my dance with indignation. It's a constant process of peeling away all that is not Love, until nothing else remains.

---

[31] Prasaad: A blessed gift.

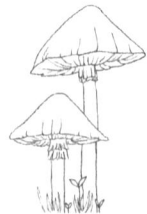

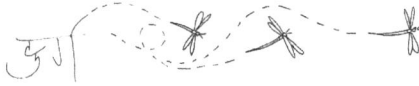

Ashram,

river,

Some wade in, sink their feet in the mud, feel the pressure of the
water rushing past their thighs and call it swimming.
Some dive in and look surprised that they are all wet.
Some, walk in, humble to the power of the water,
realize that they are not here to tame it,
to use it,
but to open to it,
let its current wash away all that is not needed,
they bow down,
float,
and allow the river to carry them to a new bank of awareness.

S.H

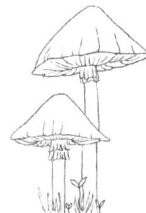

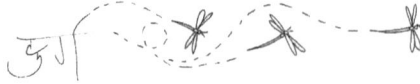

THIRTEEN

- The Illusion of Separateness

There are many paths a soul can walk, they may all look different, but in their essence they are always the same. Reality can vary, but Truth is Truth. You can eat sushi, or you can eat tacos, but in essence they are both food that is consumed with the intention of nourishing the body. Yoga, Shamanism, Christianity, Buddhism, Atheism - Your soul's palate in this lifetime will be more inclined to one over the other, and sometimes for a treat you go out and eat something different. My spirit's staple diet, in this lifetime, is Yoga. It is the framework from which I move through this world. The teachings of Yoga, Tantra and Vedanta, hold the perspective and tools to which I aspire to experience, embody and live from.

Sri Swaimiji said, "If you are looking for water, that which brings life, there is no point in digging ten holes one foot deep. Better to dig one hole ten feet deep."

As I look back over the last 18 years, since the Divine started to stir my soul from its slumber, and acutely the last 15 years, since meeting my first real teacher on the path, I can pinpoint major and minor births, stirrings, breakdowns and breakthroughs that were moments where life will never go back to the way it was. Some of these steps were large, some of them were an infinitesimal shuffle,

As our realities ebb and flow like sine waves on the ocean's surface, sometimes happy, sometimes not so, we use Sadhana, or spiritual practice, to build the muscles of the Spirit so that it becomes your ballast in a storm. Everyone at some point hits a bump in the road and comes into a varying state of crisis. It's instinctive to coast through your mundane life and when things are going well, it seems like a no brainer to keep continuing and investing your life force energy into the path of least effort, often, at the expense of your Spiritual practice. At the point of deep change or crisis however, when your whole reality has been invested into the very thing that is falling apart it can feel extremely traumatic. In my experience of sharing the teachings of Yoga and its associated philosophies, it is at this point of crisis that people turn to Yoga to help make the hurt go away. But Yoga is not a fix it science, it's more of a prevent it, and lessen the blow science. Giving you the tools and the perspective to not be as identified with the mundane for *when*, not if, it falls apart. When we are in crisis we automatically and unconsciously shift into our tried and true coping mechanisms. For some, it's tequila, for some it's the arms of a stranger, and for many others it's food that temporarily satiates and suppresses what we are feeling. I scream for Ice Cream! So many people start a Yoga practice while they are in a deep state of change only to drop it as soon as the mundane reorganizes itself into a state that is no longer immediately painful. Yet, if we are able to take these practices and let them and the teachings that support them, become a new foundation in our lives, then when our next wave of deep change comes into our reality, we have a point of consistency that we can focus on, like the point a ballerina looks at every time they finish a Fouetté turn. It keeps your balance even if you are spinning at a tremendous rate. The stream will always take the more established and carved out route upon a strong current. Our opportunity is to carve out our relationship with the Divine so that when life flows strongly in deep change, the deepest and most stable route is to be more connected to the frequencies of the Divine. Thus lessens the devastation that a flash flood can do and instead we grab our kayak and go for a wild ride.

At different times throughout the years I have had intense periods of emotional and mental pain. Excruciating bouts of perceived isolation, down to the out-right belief that I was fundamentally unlovable. They say ignorance is bliss. I say it's a bitch. Each one of these experiences has driven me to dive deeper into my enquiry of what I perceive there is, suffering and pain and what there could be, peace and contentment. And if any of it is actually real, or just two sides of a coin in the currency of time.

There is a moment though, in that cavern of crisis that a new seed has the opportunity to be planted. Not as a bandage until things can return back to 'normal', but a seed that is able to use the full fertilization of the present crap to root deep into a new level of awareness. It's experienced in the moment when one becomes a mother, out of intense pain a being of light is brought forth into this world to experience themselves from a different angle. Intense pain, be it physical, emotional or mental has the ability, with the right intension and awareness, a dash of humility and a deep breath of surrender, to be a pivotal point into which the seed immersed in the Holy in Decay[32], reaching for the light, and blossoms into a rose.

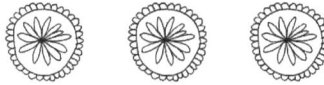

❋   ❋   ❋

2014 was one of those years. The first initial push of building Niwas was done, leaving me looking for the next endorphin rush of purpose. Instead, came a tsunami of doubt and sadness. Originating from far off shores, its origins having nothing to do with my direct experience, yet, by mere association our own beach experienced the tsunami-esque waves of emotion and destruction.

There were allegations made against people in our lineage for sexual misconduct from 30 years ago. Swamis I know who were dedicated for 20 years disrobed and took new vows of disassociation. People who had never met any party allegedly involved screamed, "burn the books!" As our own students heard

---

[32] Holy In Decay: Term credited to Martin Pretchel - The energy which takes that which has exhausted its life and empowers it to create a new. - Compost.

the news of the allegations they disassociated themselves from us. Without a word directly to me, they simply emailed everyone else we knew and said they were never speaking to us again and they never have. People lost their minds. Literally. And I had to sit with mine, which was a pit of unanswerable questions. Not really surprisingly, with a bit of research, every single lineage, religion, university, anywhere people group together basically, has had its allegations at one time or another. Not to discount the seriousness of the situation but no matter how much I listened to the allegations, through the Royal Commission that was being formally held in Australia, I couldn't find a frequency of connection. I wholeheartedly feel, with all my own experiences of questionable consent, men having power over myself and others, with my encounters of promiscuity, I am well acquainted with the cause and affect of the frequencies that bring such allegations into realities.

I called people that had closer connections with the heads of the lineage than me, both from 30 years ago, and now. They were in shock, sad and also didn't have any inclination to the validity of the allegations. People who had taken their children to both the Australian and Indian ashrams since they were babies said they had never had any ill experiences or feelings that something was amiss. Does that mean that there were things that may have happened? Sure. The fact is, I don't know. I have never experienced anything untoward in any shape or form and neither have any of the people that I reached out to to ask outright.

I prayed for guidance, which came as a dream: a huge hall filled with thousands of people chanting the 32 Names of Durga. A chant used for protection from psychic attacks. This was my sign that there was something much bigger happening here than the 3D allegations and that there was a bubble of protection in place for those that were caught in the crossfire. There were forces at work; we were all in a deep state of transformation.

We had sought blessings to build the first monks cabin back at Niwas on our previous trip to India and came home excited to fundraise for this endeavour. Alas, in the leela between intention and execution, we received an unexpected email from India. It was expressed, firmly, that our style of fundraising was out of alignment with the tradition, the teachings, and was not in right action.

Holy Shit. It was the kind of email that would make you go #Didn'tSeeItComing #WhatJustHappened #Ouch

After the 24 hours of frantic mental dancing around, "but we asked... but you said... but..." we, Paramjyoti and I, took a deep breath and wrote a letter of sincere apology. After all, it's not our intention to be out of right action. And if we are not in right action, then *we* needed to change regardless of the "buts..." Our apology was not physically responded to. India was in radio silence.

I threw my hands up in the air and said, "If Sri Swamiji wants the damn cabin, it will happen... I just don't know how." And of course, within a week, someone whom I have never met, who was an acquaintance of a friend, while over a cup of tea, spoke of a dream of a place in the woods, heard we were trying to build the cabin and cut a cheque that night for the full amount we were trying to raise in the first place.

This. This, is the blessing of *Surrender*. I could have, and my lower western mind wanted to write an email that said, "but how are we supposed to raise the funds to build the cabin if we don't fundraise?"... but that is not the point. The point is here and now, trusting, surrendering, and doing what is asked in this moment. I needed to surrender to seeming contradictions. I needed to dance in the leela of trust regardless of how the opportunity forms in this reality. These are the experiences that so clearly show me the lesson, the test, and the results of the practice. Alas, Ganesh Kutir - the remover of obstacles, was built that June.

Combine these two experiences coinciding in the same time period and you have my version of a personal spiritual crisis. After seven years of unwavering dedication, I stopped chanting my Guru mantra consistently. I didn't know what to trust. Who to believe or where to anchor my being into.

Narayana was coming up to five years old and about to start kindergarten. I realized that I had been fully on mama duty for those five years with little support from family, being that we had none in driving distance and having moved so much, we didn't have any consistent and guilt free support from friends. I'm not a person that can be outward and "on" all the time. I actually crave alone, quiet time to dive into the depths of my own creative ocean. Motherhood, for me, at least in the beginning years, didn't really allow for the energy or the opportunity or time to do this. So after five full years of "on" and a year of questioning my foundation and faith, I, well, I kinda snapped.

A local community member offered to take Narayana to the lake for a few hours to give me time to be alone. This was so rare that for the first half hour I didn't even know what to do! Should I clean? Probably. Should I read? You will never get it finished. Should I watch a movie? What a waste of time. Should I... cry? And cry I did. For no particular reason at all, I started crying, only to find out that I couldn't stop. Then I felt angry with myself that my precious 2 hours was going to be wasted in just crying. When I could be doing anything at all, all I could do was cry. No reason, no story, just exhaustion and deep despair.

So I did the only thing that I could think of in that moment that would help. I humbly, somewhat embarrassingly, emailed Sw Satsangi. I bluntly explained that I couldn't stop crying. I asked for guidance, to which came in an email not long after. "Come to Rikhia."

Sounds simple, yet, a spontaneous trip to India is anything but! Still, if your Guru says get on a plane, you get on a plane. Suddenly the winter trip for a week to Mexico in the new year, a belated honeymoon, was going out the window. There was no way we could afford to do both trips.

We chose dates, for 10 days, in a months time and then realized that not only my New Zealand passport was going to expire before the trip, but so was my permanent residence card for Canada. How to get all these things in place and an Indian visa before our trip? If She says come, then it will work out. And of course, it did.

When we arrived at Rikhia we dived into the ocean of karma yoga that precedes the Yajnas and joined the rice packing team. Happily immersed in our Seva, I was surprised on day three when I was called to see Sw Satsangi. I had never been called to her before without me asking for a meeting and my samskaras of being called to the principal's office rushed through every clammy pore of my skin in anticipation. Of course, she was lovely. She enquired on how I was feeling since my email to her and then brought up the email of reprimand about the cabin. "Did you build the cabin?" she asked. I looked up to see a sparkle in her eye and what could almost pass for the fleeting hint of knowing smile. "Yes," I replied. Then, as I looked at her, my heart screamed all the unanswered questions in the lineages disrepute. But there was an air, and an understanding of the power of words, the living reality of that which we put energy, thoughts, words into, becomes empowered. Multiple times I have now experienced that what she says manifests, like the finding of the land that is Niwas, and can only imagine the weighty responsibility of conversation. It felt as if for someone capable of such current to engage in a discussion with me, someone who it didn't directly affect and therefore was not appropriate to create that link with, would only empower the force of destruction. And yet, with all my being, on another level of awareness, I simultaneously felt an unspoken conversation, not in words, but in energy. Even though in my email I never mentioned it, I felt she knew that is why my heart hurt so much. I felt she asked me to come, to see for myself, engage with her directly, with questioning eyes, and find out what my heart would stand behind. And I knew, that I could trust her. That I might not have all the answers, but that I would one day understand a bigger picture and I would see why these things are brought forth to deal with within ourselves.

At the end of our week packing rice, we met with her again as a family. I asked her, in my usual dorky way, if she could come and have a meal with us, the greater whole ashram "us", before we left in two days. She said, "Yes, ok." That evening she came and ate in the common area where we all received meals, instead of eating privately in her kutir[33], and ate in her spot with some of the key ashramites that help to run everything smoothly. Voila, as always, she had done as she promised. The next night though, was our last night. As I left my seva to go to dinner I saw that her car was in position to be going for a drive. Often this was to come to the other compound to eat. When I got to the kitchen the kitchen yogis were in a state of frenzy trying to prepare dinner. The head of the kitchen was making her way through the people waiting and informing some long time devotees that Sw Satsangi was going to be coming for dinner, but was going to be slightly late and could they please wait to eat with her. My request from the day before flashed through my mind, but the kitchen head never came up to us so I dismissed it and went and got a plate. Narayana positioned himself between Paramjyoti and myself as we all sat crossed legged on the second mat back eating a delicious treat of "street food" consisting of spicy beans and the buns that Paramjyoti had himself made for dinner. I sat and chatted with another karma sannyasin about the day's events and watched as the kitchen staff set up Sw Satsangi's mat and the place settings for her guests a little ways in front of the rest of the mats.

As I'm scoffing down my yummy dinner, I see two feet in front of my plate. Just like in the movies I slowly pan up to see that

---

[33] Kutir: Small dwelling

it is Sw Satsangi standing in front of me with her hands on her hips. "I said I was going to come and eat with you but you have started without me," she proclaimed as I nearly spat out my mouthful of food. "Ah, the kitchen informed all your guests and they didn't say anything to me, so I figured you would eat with the VIP's and... I can have seconds?" She seemed to look around in the debate of what to do, go and sit where they had put her setting and ask us to come up? Or to let us stay there and eat and go and eat with the others. Suddenly, she plopped herself down on the first row of mats facing me and gestured that she would sit there for dinner. Everyone in the first row, who were rightly facing the opposite direction to her, got up and skedaddled. Leaving Sw Satsangi to be the only one on the mat.

The seating team sprung into unfamiliar territory and moved Sw Satsangi's setting to in front of her, and proceeded to put the other place settings around us. The VIP's and other head Swami's used to eating with her looked confused and unsure of what to do. She gestured to the group of confused looking guests to sit next to us, some on the first mat, and some on the second and we all preceded to eat, some of us, for a second helping.

You would think that when you are seated with a Master, a Guru, for dinner that you would have some deep philosophical conversation about Vedanta, or the world, or the Gita and so forth. Well, not in my experience anyway, the conversation was light and jovial. Sw Satsangi spoke of childhood experiences of eating this exact "street food" when she was growing up. How she drinks lemon and water rather than tea in the morning and we chatted about the joys of eating an artichoke with garlic butter. How the petals of the artichoke really are just a vehicle for spooning garlic butter as you make your way to the heart of the flower.

The gentleman eating with us who had sponsored the dinner asked if it was too spicy for the westerners. To which we replied that it was very tasty and not too hot. Suddenly the air changed and

I felt the need to apologize again for eating before she arrived. "I really thought you were just going to eat with the VIP's," I offered. "Are you not a VIP?" she exclaimed in front of everyone. "Ah, no. No I'm not," I said embarrassed and awkward. "Everyone here is a VIP. Everyone here holds the same place in my heart, there are no favourites, no one is more important than the others." Now I started to burn from the inside out, blushing to the tune of a summer ripe tomato. "Wow, it's getting really hot in here," I said fanning myself with my hand. "This is the colour the westerners go when the food is too spicy." I told the gentleman who had offered the food. Everyone laughed, including Sw Satsangi, which is always a Divine sight.

The laughter and the blushing seemed to peel away my formal awkwardness and made me relax a little. Then, as Sw Satsangi lent forward to take a bite of her meal, she tilted her head up and looked me in the eye. It may have been a few seconds, one second even, but in that moment, for me, time completely stopped. As she looked me in the eye I was transfixed. Frozen as I felt a new energy wash over me. In the moment I was completely conscious that I was experiencing something that is called Shakti Path. A transmission of energy from Guru to someone that is an offering of blessings, of support on an energetic level. I felt that this is what we had physically gotten on the plane and flown to the other side of the world. This glimpse of the beyond in the flash of an eye.

Suddenly, Sw. Satsangi stood up, smiled, said, "Namo Narayana," and walked away having simply finished her meal. I, on the other hand, sat there forever changed.

The next morning I went to Guru Puja before we were to leave on the train Canada bound. As I sat there, I was calm. I would not say joyful, but no longer distressed as I was before we came to India. I was emotionally neutral and sat with gratitude in my heart as we chanted. As we got to the fourth to last verse of the chant, out of nowhere, tears started to stream from my eyes. I was taken aback by this spontaneous shift in my energy body and closed my eyes. When I did, BOOM, a flash of My Guru's beloved face, in the same look as during the look she had given me the evening before. A flash of thought, *You need to bless your mala,* startled me, quickly followed by, *Oh Shivani, your ego of needing more, needing another interaction, needing something special. It's ridiculous. You have everything you need. She has given you everything, now go and do something with it.* OK, I thought, if I see her without any doing on my part, I will ask her if she will bless my mala, the same one she had given me during my initiation seven years prior, and if I don't see her I will take it as my fanciful mind playing tricks. After the Puja had finished we did the usual circling of Sri Swamiji's Samadhi sthal and I headed over to Hanuman for blessings to jump the ocean and then to Durga for her protection. As I stepped down to the spot where Ma Durga's murti[34] sits, Sw Satsangiji was standing outside of her house, next to the fence, watching me with her hand out waiting for my mala. I don't know why I keep feeling surprised by these moments. In one smooth motion I removed the mala from my neck, rolled my eyes and had the smile on my face that resembles Carlton's dance on the Fresh Prince of Bel Air.

There were no words needed, everything in our short trip had been communicated in abundance and with so much kindness. A simple "Namo Narayana" was offered and to Canada we returned.

A few weeks later we were blessed by having our dear friends Salvatore and Rebecca Zambito come and stay with us. The most beautiful gift of all that year was that Salvatore, a scholar of Patanjali's Yoga Sutras and practitioner for over 40 years sat and answered all of my questions about the Great White Brotherhood. It truly felt like a gift from Sri Swamiji to have the answers offered to me in a way that I could understand. As Salvatore explained to me the different processes of Initiations at different levels of

---

[34] Murti: Statue

consciousness, I could not help but wonder if this information was being made available to me then as an answer to a prayer of wanting to understand the bigger picture of the events of that year and how the purification for the lineage as a whole that year was quite possibly connected to this level of Initiation.

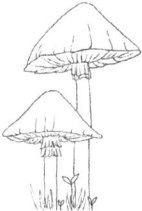

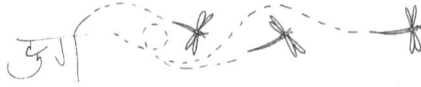

FOURTEEN

- A Prayer and a Promise part two

"Modernity's seemingly bottomless addiction to an endless pursuit of recreation, substances (legal or not), TV, or religious or scientific promises of another more anesthetized world, of having to constantly "escape" or "get away" from an everyday life of dead, demythologized stuff, and a daily insignificance in a scheme-less, unstirred whole is fast creating an anti-existence based on forgetting instead of remembering, which, if it doesn't first kill the viability of the holy ground we need to live on by compromising the diverse "Seed Heart" in its flight of escape, we will someday not have enough reality left here on earth in our bodies to remember, much less anything to remember it with; the muscle and its reason for existing would atrophy simultaneously."

Martin Prechtel[35],

Sometimes as we start to awaken to an expanded perspective of reality, of who we are, why we are here and the whole point of this delicious dance called life, we start to Re-member things in a new light. Literally. We start to engage with the present in a way that lets the past be an adorning of our souls, reflecting and refracting light to create beauty, rather than being old socks we stuff in a suitcase and lug around with us. When past, present and future all become tangible threads weaving the cloth we are wrapped in, in the here and now, we can soften our skin into Divinities embrace and move through this world with our feet on the ground, our head in the clouds and one ear on the whispers the beings unseen offer unconditionally.

---

[35] *from the The Unlikely Peace at Cuchumaquic.*

In Re-membering we expand, and we liberate the tiny box our minds hold on to for dear life. Without realizing that the life that it encases, is not really living at all. Not to our fullest potential anyway. The action alone of acknowledging and taking responsibility for the guided cage we perceive our lives from, invokes enough frequency to liberate patterns held so dear and for far too long. Then to take that seed of new found potential, and lay it at the feet of the Divine as a flower of surrender is truly, an act of Praise for life and of Gratitude for the opportunity of a beating heart in a human body.

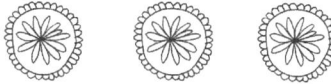

2015 heralded the 25th year since Sri Swamiji stepped onto the land I know and love as Rikhia. We travelled to the Ashram for our yearly seva, with my dear friend Om Shanti and her son Ty. Narayana, now six, flitted between helping us with our seva and playing with all the other kids in the Ashram. It was the biggest Yajnas in terms of Daan, or giving, that I had ever seen. Clothes and schoolbags, thousands upon thousands of village bags bursting at the seams with Love in the manifested forms of saris, sweaters, prasaad, rice, and all of the other essential items that the local people utilize in their day to day life.

There were not two Yajnas this year but three, with no gaps in between them, just go, go, go, give, give, give, 4am til 9pm each day. It was amazing, awe-inspiring, and grueling. Yet, amongst the intensity of it all there was such a wonderful underlying joy and purpose to the whole event. People from all over the world come to this, different cultures, ages and languages, all showing up to be part of the Sankalpa or resolve of a Paramahansa, our beloved Sri Swamiji. To uplift the community, the world, through this ancient offering by worshiping the Divine forms and formless aspects of Devi, Shiva and Agni or fire. It's a humbling experience and an honour to be a part of the dance.

That being said, the purpose of intense Karma yoga is to create an opportunity for oneself to change, for inner transformation. And inner transformation only comes when the ego is tired. When it can no longer hold its facade to the world, the dam breaks and all the stagnant energy of ignorance rushes forward frantically seeking a path home to the Divine arms of the Ocean. The long hours of a Yajna, the mental and physical effort and the intensity of the Puja that is happening, makes one ripe for such fatigue, which means that at some point, everyone loses their composure and gets triggered into their patterns of negativity. Myself included.

I had been thoroughly seated in joy and purpose for the first Yajnas. Embracing my sankalpa of "running the cobbles," where I don't wear shoes during the Yajnas. It's purely my thing, not an ashram thing, but I found with the fast pace of my duty and the often urgency of requests, if I have to constantly look for my shoes every time I go in and out of a building then I find I loose my mental thread and one pointed focus on the seva at hand. It distracts me from my duty, so I decided to strengthen my feet enough to be able to run, literally, on the cobbled path, moving as fast as I could all the while dodging the cobbles that stick up and bite your big toe if you are not paying attention. If I was tired, or perturbed by something, or my feet were sore that day, I would sometimes imagine Sri Swamiji walking ahead of me on the path, my eyes focusing only on his feet and the bottom of his dhoti. I'd mutter to myself over and over,

"All I see is your feet, All I hear is the Name."

Every time I conjured this image I no longer felt my sore feet, or had an emotional attachment to whatever was perturbing me. The frequency of my mind had re-orientated my physical perception allowing me to focus purely on the task at hand pouring heart and soul to each action only for the success of His sankalpa[36].

During the last Yajna, the four days of Shiva worship, called Yog Poornima, my cup was full and my opportunity for change boiled to the surface like a volcano from my absolute depths.

I could feel my nervous system getting over strung like the string of a violin, about to snap and scar the person currently winding it at any moment. It was early afternoon so there was a lull in our duty and I asked to be excused for not feeling well. I retreated to my room hoping that I could quell my outburst into a polite transformation of a few tears and a good self talking to. But when I got back to my room there was a loud speaker blasting the audio from what was happening on stage. Without the context of being able to see the visual story unfolding and without knowing Hindi, I wasn't unable to appreciate or comprehend the sounds pouring into my room. And without a current context to put it into, it threw me into a visceral reliving of all my memories of isolation, hearing others in extreme mental and emotional pain without being able to help, entrapment, powerlessness and abandonment. I couldn't make the sound stop and I didn't feel well enough to leave my room, nor would I have anywhere to go if I did. I had to just sit there, my knees tucked under my chin with my hands over my ears and ride out what my filters translated to be a terrible, vicious argument between two people. I was catapulted into emotionally being a six year old listening to parents scream at each other. As I sat there trying to hide from the sound waves of voices who didn't know their power to hurt, the festering heat of an infected wound my soul had carried for far too long started to sweat from every pore of my skin. The stories of being abandoned and rejected by the

---

36 Sankalpa: Intention of manifestation and embodiment.

masculine, of being lied to by the feminine, of not being able to trust or anchor into anything for fear of the rug being pulled from underneath me, poured forth from me and projected over the only form of the masculine that could hold my ignorance for what it was worth. Sri Swamiji. I started to feel that all the moments in childhood when I didn't feel safe, when I couldn't feel the Divine protecting me, when my beloved Grandfather died, when I experienced the masculine of push me pull you, I want you, but I don't want YOU, instability of my faith in 2014, and with the questioning of a child who simply can't comprehend why adults make such painful decisions, burst forth through tears and snot. "Why did you leave me?" "Why were you not there?" "Why are you not here now!?"

And in that moment, I cried out as the victim. From the depths of agony, the pain of my own ignorance, of the forgetting of my true nature, I was hit with a frequency of scolding so forceful it stopped my tears midway down my face. The energy was of Shiva, no nonsense scolding, not of violence, of utter purity and strength pierced into me.

"You think that I have left YOU, but I can't! You are a fool! It is your own wounding that makes you feel this! YOU are creating this feeling! It is YOU who has disconnected, YOU who has stopped fully trusting, YOU who has stopped practicing your mantra faithfully. It is YOU who is waiting for the bad things to happen so that you can say, 'I told you so.' I have committed to you, as you have to me, we are karmically bound. If you can't feel me with you that is YOUR fault, that is your doing, you have disconnected. I cannot leave you, I am here, always."

Sitting there, the audio still blasting into my room but no longer holding my attention, I was catapulted into a memory. Of me, showing up to the Ashram with a Prayer and A Promise in 2007. A prayer for a husband of my equal and a child to share this life with. A promise to surrender, to offer every breath from that moment in service to the light that Sri Swamiji embodied. And I saw myself from across the Puja area. I was dressed all in white, on my hands and knees washing the marble Puja floor in front of Shiva. I saw Sri Swamiji standing, hands on his hips, just a few feet away from me, flanked by Sw Niranjan, and by Sw Satsangi. And I saw, in that moment, a beam of light, a rippling of sound waves, of energy, transfer from me to Sri Swamiji, and from Sri Swamiji to me. I consciously remembered this moment in 2007, but I was not aware back then that this was the moment that my prayer and promise and been solidified through a type of initiation. In hindsight, as I was being shown now, this was the moment I was born into this life.

As I realized this, saw the memory being shown, I recognized the actions that I needed to take to let go of this next layer of my onion. I felt all the toxic memories surge through my system in one volcanic eruption of lunch. I cried, I threw up, and I cried some more. But these tears were not tears for the past, they were a deep grieving of the soul who realizes the weight and burden of pain they have carried for so long through their own ignorance, as the light of Remembrance of who they truly are starts to shine through the cracks. The tears kept flowing, but they shifted from tears of grief and acknowledgement, to tears of Gratitude for this life and opportunities of the present. For over 24 hours my body re-orientated itself on every level. I slept, I purged, I lay on my bed and bathed in the Mantras of Shiva. But there was no suffering or feeling of being ill, just of deep, deep, fatigue as I let go of that which was no longer serving me and an opening up
to a new foundation of Trust at the depths of my
soul.

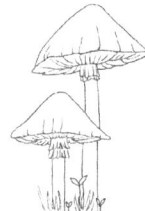

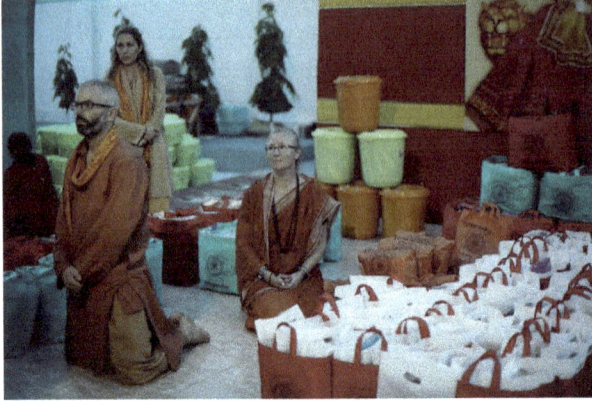

The last time I wore a Sari. 2016 on the last day of the Sat Chandi Maha Yajna.

I'd love like

I'm not scared,

Give when it's not fair,

Live life for another,

Take time for a brother,

Fight for the weak ones,

Speak out for freedom,

Find faith in the battle,

Stand tall but above it all,

Fix my eyes on you...

Fix My Eyes
For King & Country

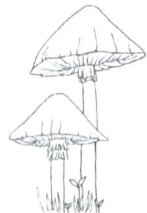

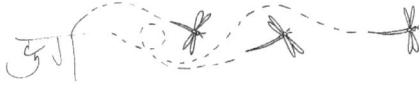

EPILOGUE

Come, let us listen,
To the whispers suspended between the here and now
The ones we will only fully understand,
In the silence of tomorrow.

The soul is on a journey, from ignorance and inertia to Re-membering an awareness so complete it no longer believes it is separate from the light. The further refined your perception becomes, as you have stilled your inner distractions and turbulence, the more time is spent in a deep state of listening. You start to feel or perceive information on a much more subtle level; hear what is said between words, feeling the frequencies of light emanating from everything, from a person to a tree, bird to a rock. Each interaction becomes a silent awareness of interconnectivity. Each place you focus your outward senses on comes a witnessing of the weaving of light on all levels of your being. Suddenly you become aware, you Re-member your being as an interconnected facet of the whole. And in that interconnectivity the light you weave, the songs you entertain dancing with, ripple and affect every blade of grass as it emanates out from you. Suddenly listening and dancing in light is a more focused way and more complete way of moving through your existence. From this place, in the seat of this awareness, each verbal word uttered speaks volumes to those who can hear, each look shines light on those who can see, each touch changes forever the heart of those who dare to feel.

"Faith is the greatest asset of man's personality.
If you have faith, you have everything."
Paramahansa Satyananda Saraswati

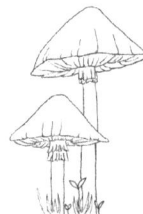

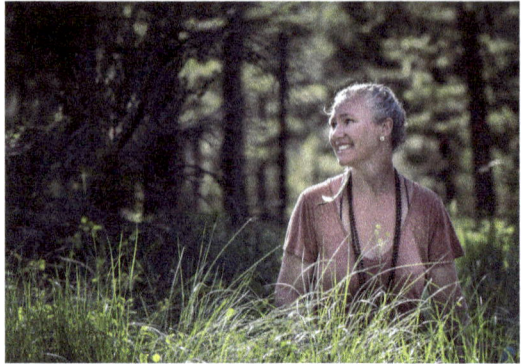

About Shivani,

Shivani Howe is the founder of the Ishtadev Niwas Ashram located at the foothills of both the Rocky and Purcell Mountains in Southeast British Columbia, Canada. She is deeply connected to the natural world and is also the co-owner operator of Ishtadev Niwas Farm where she lives, dreams and works with her husband Paramjyoti, son Narayana and a variety of animals including but not limited to alpacas, dogs, chickens, goats, sheep, cats and ducks.

In 2001, Shivani was challenged with a painful and 'incurable' disease and decided to take a new approach to life. This is when she discovered the ancient philosophy of Yoga. The New Zealand native not only healed her endometriosis, but brought harmony to her life and body, by unraveling the stresses of her illness from its source.

Since then Shivani has completed over a thousand hours of intensive Yoga training and is a certified E-RYT 500 Yoga teacher and teacher trainer. Guided by her own personal experiences Shivani's intuition and expertise is invaluable as she assists others to discover their own truths and align themselves with their highest potential.

Shivani finds much joy in facilitating retreats and classes, supporting her students in discovering new ways of living and being. Yet her greatest joy is found listening to the birds sing, talking with the trees, watching the garden grow and playing with and learning from her son, her greatest teacher.

About Ishtadev Niwas Ashram

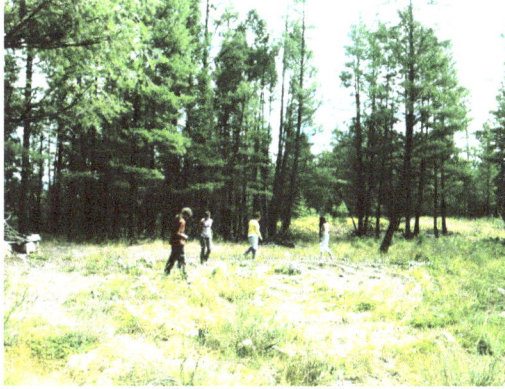

Yoga . Philosophy . Yoga Ecology

At Ishtadev Niwas, we believe that the entire Universe is interconnected. As individuals living in a complicated world, each of our actions has an effect on everything around us. The choices we make, our actions, our thoughts, all emit energy that leads us toward peace, or toward chaos.

Founded and run by the Living Yoga Society (2010), Ishtadev Niwas is an Ashram and Yoga Centre designed to guide people of all ages toward a better understanding of their inner dynamic. Our courses and classes teach people how to apply the principles of Vedic and Tantric philosophies to the modern Western lifestyle, rooted in the traditional 5 paths of Yoga and centering around Yoga Ecology, Ashram Life, and the science of Karma Yoga. We support people with tools to assist their exploration of their inner self, the Universe as a whole, and techniques for living in harmony with all the day-to-day challenges that everyone must face.

We believe that Yoga is not something you practice, it's something you Live.

An individual's journey through the Universe is greatly aided by a deep understanding of their own role, and the steady balance of their emotional, financial, intellectual and spiritual lives. From the health of the body to the health of the planet, the health of the mind to the healing of the soul, 'Niwas guides people on the path toward improving themselves, and thereby improving the world around them. This is what Yoga Ecology is all about.

Come join us at Ishtadev Niwas, an Ashram embodying the ancient philosophy and teachings of Yoga through every day life. Situated in the foothills of the pristine Purcell Mountains in beautiful British Columbia, Ishtadev Niwas is a sacred place of healing and transformation. Cleanse and purify your mind, body and Spirit and experience living in conscious community, surrounded by breathtaking mountain views.

For more information check out
www.ishtadevniwas.ca

www.ingramcontent.com/pod-product-compliance
Lightning Source LLC
Chambersburg PA
CBHW050733030426
42336CB00012B/1546